Revitalization: Explorations in World Christian Movements

This volume is published in collaboration with the Center for the Study of World Christian Revitalization Movements, a cooperative initiative of Asbury Theological Seminary faculty. Building on the work of the previous Wesleyan/Holiness Studies Center at the Seminary, the Center provides a focus for research in the Wesleyan Holiness and related Christian renewal movements, including Pietism and Pentecostal movements, which have had a world impact. The research seeks to develop analytical models of these movements, including their biblical and theological assessment. Using an interdisciplinary approach, the Center bridges relevant discourses in several areas in order to gain insights for effective Christian mission. It recognizes the need for conducting research that combines insights from the history of evangelical renewal and movements with anthropological and religious studies literature on revitalization movements. It networks with similar research centers around the world, in addition to sponsoring its own research projects.

Joanna Cruickshank's study of the theme of suffering in the hymns of Charles Wesley, a subject considered distasteful to many nineteenth-century Methodists, reveals Wesley's deeply pastoral exploration of a question of enduring theological significance. It also illuminates a central aspect of early Methodist culture, which had implications for Methodist responses to issues such as the abolition of slavery, the role of women, missionary activity and the existence of hell. Charles Wesley's success in probing the depths of human pathos with the redemptive message of Christianity reveals much about why primitive Methodism represented a movement of depth and practical efficacy to so many who were overlooked by the conventional religious practices of that day. As such, it represents an important resource for scholars as well as persons interested in the sources of early modern religious awakenings. Hence, this volume, a seminal study of Charles Wesley, is also congruent with the mission of the Center and addresses its research objectives.

J. Steven O'Malley, Director
Center for the Study of World Christian Revitalization Movements
Asbury Theological Seminary

Pain, Passion and Faith

Revisiting the Place of Charles Wesley in Early Methodism

Joanna Cruickshank

Revitalization: Explorations in World Christian Movements
Pietist and Wesleyan Studies, No. 31

THE SCARECROW PRESS, INC.
Lanham • Toronto • Plymouth, UK
and
The Center for the Study of World Christian Revitalization Movements
2009

Published by Scarecrow Press, Inc.
A wholly owned subsidiary of The Rowman & Littlefield Publishing Group, Inc.
4501 Forbes Boulevard, Suite 200, Lanham, Maryland 20706
http://www.scarecrowpress.com

Estover Road, Plymouth PL6 7PY, United Kingdom

British Library Cataloguing in Publication Information Available

Library of Congress Cataloging-in-Publication Data

Cruickshank, Joanna, 1974–
Pain, passion and faith : revisiting the place of Charles Wesley in early Methodism / Joanna Cruickshank.
p. cm. — (Pietist and Wesleyan studies ; no. 31) (Revitalization: explorations in world Christian movements)
Includes bibliographical references and index.
ISBN 978-0-8108-6154-1 (pbk. : alk. paper) — ISBN 978-0-8108-7398-8 (ebook)
1. Suffering—Religious aspects—Christianity. 2. Pain—Religious aspects—Christianity. 3. Methodist Church—Hymns—History and criticism. 4. Wesley, Charles, 1707–1788. 5. Methodist Church—Doctrines. I. Title.
BT732.7.C78 2009
287.092—dc22 2009027101

™ The paper used in this publication meets the minimum requirements of American National Standard for Information Sciences—Permanence of Paper for Printed Library Materials, ANSI/NISO Z39.48-1992.

Printed in the United States of America

Contents

Editor's Preface

This volume introduces contemporary scholars and admirers of the vast hymnody of Charles Wesley, brother of the founder of Methodism in eighteenth-century England, to the definitive study of the role of pain and suffering in the corpus of his hymnody. Joanna Cruickshank documents how this issue became a major point of disagreement between the two famous Wesley brothers, Charles and John. It also offers an important contribution to our understanding of the historical development of Christian responses to suffering. Noting that thousands of Wesley's hymns focused on the experience of overwhelming pain, her study examines these in depth. Some, she notes, portrayed the sacrificial agonies of Jesus, while others depicted the afflictions of individual Christians in experiences as diverse as persecution, smallpox and bereavement. A topic commonly avoided in the history of Methodism, and even by his influential brother, John Wesley, it is here retrieved as constituting a theme of seminal importance to early Methodism, understood as a revival movement.

One typically identifies the theme of pain and suffering with the literature of German Pietism. The emphasis on human suffering was considered distasteful by many, and few of these hymns were reproduced in nineteenth-century hymnbooks. However, we also know that Charles, in different ways from his brother John, had significant contacts with Halle Pietism as well as the Moravians. Hence, it may be that this theme represents one of the connecting links that illumine the affinity that existed between Pietism and early Methodism. Such a linkage surely commends this study as one appropriate to the *Pietist and Wesleyan Studies* sub-series, offered here within the series concerned with explorations in world Christian revitalization movements.

J. Steven O'Malley, Series Editor

Acknowledgments

Like Charles Wesley, I am "of a social temper," and have been much blessed by the companionship and support of many people while writing this book. The School of Historical Studies at the University of Melbourne provided a collegial environment in which to work on this project. David Philips, whose untimely death has deprived the historical community of a fine scholar, provided encouraging and insightful supervision of the doctoral research from which this book arises. Paul Nicholls also provided very helpful and often hilarious comments on my work. More recently, I have appreciated the opportunity of working with Patricia Grimshaw, whose enthusiasm and generosity have been a great gift. Juliet Flesch, Tim Jones, Rob McArthur, Rick Clapton and Kelly Chaves are among many colleagues who have shared good conversation and not-so-good coffee with me over the years. Erica Mehrtens and her fellow administrative staff have competently and cheerfully made things happen. During the final stages of preparing the manuscript, my new colleagues in the School of History, Heritage and Society at Deakin University have been welcoming and supportive.

Throughout this project, I have been overwhelmed by the generosity of Methodist scholars around the world. Gareth Lloyd at the John Rylands University Library in Manchester has been unfailingly helpful as a guide to Charles Wesley and the world of English Methodism. Tom Albin kindly gave me access to his transcripts of Methodist letters and Kenneth Newport was similarly generous with his transcript of Charles Wesley's journal. Jeremy Gregory, David Hempton and Phyllis Mack have all made helpful comments on my ideas about Charles Wesley and early Methodism.

In bringing the book to publication, I have been very grateful to Randy Maddox for his encouragement to publish; to J. Steven O'Malley and his colleagues on the editorial committee of the *Pietist and Wesleyan Studies* series for their assistance; and to April Snider at Scarecrow Press for her patient support in the task of producing the manuscript.

Many friends and family members have supported me through the process of completing this book. My friend Michelle Charis knows more about both suffering and being sympathetic than most, and has been a constant encouragement. My parents, Peter and Jenny Richardson, and wonderful family, both Richardsons and Cruickshanks, have reminded me of what really matters. Naomi Richardson has been a patient listener and wise friend. Most of all, I am grateful to my husband, Andrew, who has supported me wholeheartedly in this as in everything.

David and Betty Walker, my grandparents, both died while I was working on this project. They were warm hearted Christian believers who loved Charles Wesley's hymns, deeply valued intellectual enquiry and prayed that their grandchildren would be peacemakers in a violent world. I miss them very much and I dedicate this book to them.

Quotations of documents from the Methodist Archives and Research Centre are included by courtesy of the University Librarian and Director, the John Rylands University Library, The University of Manchester. An early version of Chapter Three was published as "'Appear as Crucified for Me': Sight, Suffering and Spiritual Transformation in the Hymns of Charles Wesley," *Journal of Religious History* 30, no. 3 (2006). Portions of Chapter Six appeared as "'The Suffering Members Sympathize': Constructing the Sympathetic Self in the Hymns of Charles Wesley," in *Charles Wesley: Life, Literature and Legacy*, edited by Kenneth Newport and Ted Campbell (Peterborough: Epworth Press, 2007).

Publication of this work was assisted by a publication grant from the University of Melbourne.

Abbreviations

BEW	*The Bicentennial Edition of the Works of John Wesley*
CWJ	*Journal of Charles Wesley* (ed. Thomas Jackson)
HSP	*Hymns and Sacred Poems*
HTTP	*Hymns for Times of Trouble and Persecution*
HUF	*Hymns for the Use of Families*
PCM	*Prayers for Condemned Malefactors*
PW	*The Poetical Works of John and Charles Wesley*
SHSPHS	*Short Hymns on Select Passages of Holy Scripture*
UP	*The Unpublished Works of Charles Wesley*

Unless otherwise indicated, manuscript citations are from the Methodist Archive and Research Centre, John Rylands University Library, Manchester. Because of the large number of quotations in the text, spelling and punctuation have been modernized.

Introduction

Pain, Passion and Christian Faith

In July 1758 Charles Wesley, Methodist preacher and poet, received a letter describing a mastectomy recently performed upon a Methodist woman. Titled "An account of Mrs. Davis's behavior during the operation of her breast being cut out," it was written by a woman who had been present during the operation. She wrote of Mrs. Davis:

> When the inside of her breast was taken out she asked, if they had done cutting; I answered yes, and some thread being called for, she immediately said there is some in my work basket on the table: while they sewed up the blood vessel, she said this pain is very great, she called on the Lord to strengthen her and said I'm faint.[1]

The thought of the pain that Mrs. Davis must have endured during this operation is, at least to the reader accustomed to the comforts of anesthesia and analgesics, horrifying. This matter-of-fact account, and the emotional response it engenders, raises the immediate question: how did men and women of the eighteenth century endure suffering such as this?

The very existence of this account suggests that this question was important to the eighteenth-century people who wrote and read these words as well. The anonymous writer who composed this record, and sent it to Charles Wesley, did so on the assumption that he would be interested in this detailed description of one individual's suffering. The emphasis in the title of the letter, on Mrs. Davis's "behavior," suggests that what was of particular interest was the individual's response to suffering. Mrs. Davis's behavior in the crucible of physical agony was of profound spiritual concern. This account points to the central questions that this study seeks to answer. Why did suffering matter to Wesley and his fellow Methodists? What shaped their responses to life's physical and emotional pain? How did their understanding of suffering reflect or resist attitudes to suffering within the wider cultural context of eighteenth-century England?[2]

I address these questions by examining the way that the experience of suffering is constructed in a particular set of early Methodist texts: the hymns of Charles Wesley. Among Wesley's thousands of hymns are many that explore in great detail the meaning of pain, and the appropriate Christian responses to it. Identifying the construction of suffering in these works does not reveal exactly how early Methodists responded to suffering, but it does illuminate these responses. Through their focused exploration of the meaning of suffering, Wesley's hymns draw our attention to language, narratives and theological frameworks through which Methodists could interpret, describe and manage painful experiences. Studying these elements within Wesley's hymns allows us to understand more clearly the many descriptions and discussions of suffering that appear in the letters, journals and life narratives of "ordinary" English Methodists of the same period.

As they sang or read Wesley's hymns, Methodists were encouraged to adopt a distinctive approach to suffering, an approach that drew upon long-standing elements within Christian traditions as well as new patterns in eighteenth-century English culture. Ultimately, however, it was unusual in relation to both Protestant Christianity and the contemporary context. Examining this approach will lead us to revisit the place that Charles Wesley and his hymns held within early Methodism. More broadly, it will illuminate the culture of early Methodism and its complicated relationship to its eighteenth-century English context.

The term "suffering" is central to this book, and requires further definition. The development of cultural history has meant an increased interest in analyzing the meanings that different individuals and cultures have given to pain and suffering.[3] While such works often refer to pain and suffering, few historians have concerned themselves with distinguishing between the two terms. This does not mean that these terms have simple or uncontested meanings. Both terms are used to describe unpleasant sensation, but in common usage the distinction between pain and suffering is unclear.[4]

In modern medicine, the two are often distinguished in terms of professional specialties. While physical pain is seen as the business of the physician, "distress or misery in the wider sense" is understood as a matter for clergy, friends and psychotherapists.[5] However, this type of distinction, which identifies pain as a matter of the body and suffering as a matter of the spirit or mind, is inadequate. It relies on a flawed notion that pain can be divided into two discrete categories of "physical" and "mental" pain. For the historian, studying cultures with very different conceptions of the relationship between mind or spirit and body, such a simple distinction may be completely misleading. And, apart from the wider philosophical questions about mind and body that such a distinction raises, pain and suffering are often used as overlapping or interchangeable concepts.

In his history of suffering, Joseph Amato calls our attention to the way in which pain is usually used to talk about specific or localized sensation, whereas suffering implies totality of some sort. Suffering, he has suggested, is a more comprehensive experience than pain, and the term rightly describes "a general condition, person, group or society." For this reason, we do not "speak of the many sufferings of a person's pain, whereas we commonly speak of suffering as if it is composed of many pains."[6] Amato's definition is useful because it clarifies the significance of suffering for the individual or the group. Suffering is never trivial in nature, but implies pain or pains that to some extent engulf those experiencing them. For this reason, suffering may challenge any attempts to explain or describe.[7] While suffering almost always contains some physical element, however, it may not entirely or even largely be a matter of physical pain: experiences such as grief, loneliness and fear may certainly be described as suffering. This explanation, which emphasizes the overwhelming nature of the experience of suffering, is reflected in Wesley's use of the term and therefore in my analysis. This book focuses on experiences of pain – emotional, physical or spiritual – that overwhelm (or threaten to overwhelm) the individual or group.

This definition does, however, leave a number of questions unanswered. Who determines that a certain experience will be defined as "suffering"? What are the respective roles of culture, the individual or the "expert" in this process of definition? Such questions draw attention to the constructed nature of the experience of suffering: it does not simply happen to people, but is created both by what happens and by how they make sense of it.[8] The study of suffering, like that of pain of all kinds, requires an awareness of the historical and cultural contexts in which individuals experience and interpret the hardships they encounter.

In using the term "construction," I am not implying a "hard constructionist" view of experience, which assumes that "there is no limit to the extent to which personal feelings are socially, locally, culturally constructed."[9] I affirm historian D. Bruce Hindmarsh's contention, in relation to early evangelical conversion narratives, that converts understood themselves to be discovering, rather than constructing, their religious experiences.[10] Rather, my use of this language points to the role of the hymns in shaping the experience and expression of suffering. This study is not concerned primarily with the individual experiences of suffering that early Methodists endured, but with the hymns as a means of making sense and spiritual use of that suffering. As will be seen, both Charles Wesley and those who used the hymns understood them as a tool for this purpose.

The argument that the experience of suffering had particular importance for early Methodists is not new. Famously, the Marxist historian E. P. Thompson argued that Methodist culture gave an unhealthy centrality to suffering, both in its focus on the sufferings of Christ and in its conviction of the value of suffering for the soul. In typically biting style, Thompson contended:

> It is difficult to conceive of a more essential disorganization of human life, a pollution of the sources of spontaneity bound to reflect itself in every aspect of personality. Since joy was associated with sin and guilt, and pain (Christ's wounds) with goodness and love, so every impulse became twisted into the reverse...To labour and to sorrow was to find pleasure, and masochism was 'Love'.[11]

It is significant that although Thompson mentioned Charles Wesley only in passing, he based this argument largely on an analysis of the hymnody of Methodism and most of the hymns he quoted as evidence were written by Charles.[12]

My analysis supports Thompson's contention that suffering was a central feature of both Charles Wesley's hymns and early Methodist culture. This book examines in much more detail, however, the construction of suffering in the hymns. We will also consider the relationship between the hymns and the culture of early Methodism and the relationship between the construction of suffering in the hymns and changing understandings of suffering in eighteenth-century England.

In doing so, this study contributes to the neglected task of historicizing Charles Wesley and his hymns. Few scholars have followed E. P. Thompson's lead in exploring the connections between Charles Wesley, his hymns and his broader historical context. A quick survey of the standard histories of eighteenth-century England will show the scarcity of his name in most indexes. Conversely, while Charles has been the focus of a growing number of studies by scholars of Methodism, few of these have looked closely at the historical context in which he lived and worked, beyond the theological and literary discourses and ecclesiastical politics of his time.

As the following chapters note, a number of biographies exist that examine Charles's personality, relationships and activities.[13] Many of these biographies have, however, been limited as historical works by a lack of access to relevant primary sources and a preoccupation with didactic or devotional concerns. Our knowledge of Charles's role and significance within the Methodist movement has recently taken a quantum leap forward, with the publication of Gareth Lloyd's meticulously researched book, *Charles Wesley and the Struggle for Methodist Identity*.[14] Charles Wesley has also received attention from theologians, who have identified the doctrinal framework, distinctiveness and sources of his hymns.[15] Literary scholars have been the most attentive to the cultural context of Charles's writings, and scholars like Frank Baker, J. R. Watson, Donald Davie and Janet Todd have produced valuable insights into his work, drawing on literary discourses of the time.[16] However, as Jeremy Gregory has concluded in a recent essay, the challenge remains for historians to place Charles Wesley within the many rich and insightful interpretations of eighteenth-century culture and society that recent scholarship has produced.[17]

This book contributes to the process of historicizing Charles Wesley. It begins by revisiting Charles Wesley's life and writings, considering the personal context within which the hymns were written. In the second chapter, the hymns themselves are revisited, through an analysis of their cultural function. This chapter examines the historical context of the genre of "hymn" within which Wesley wrote, as well as the hymns themselves and Wesley's own use of them. This provides an approach for my reading of the hymns throughout the book as a whole.

The remainder of the book focuses on the construction of suffering in the hymns. The third chapter examines Wesley's portrayal of the suffering of Christ, a central topic in many of his hymns, and the basis of much of his interpretation of the meaning of pain. Chapters Four and Five consider Wesley's description of the place of suffering within Christian life, focusing on his construction of the overarching narrative of Christian life, and his depiction of the appropriate management of specific experiences of suffering in the process of sanctification. Finally, Chapter Six moves from the individual to the community, examining Wesley's depiction of the role of suffering in community formation.

Life in eighteenth-century England produced many agonizing experiences such as that endured by Mrs. Davis "while having her breast cut out." The hymns of Charles Wesley provided Methodists with a means of interpreting these sufferings as part of God's work in their lives. In doing so, they gave suffering a central place in the Christian life. The resulting construction of the normative Christian experience had consequences for Methodist understandings of God, the self, Christian fellowship and society.

Notes

1. "An account of Mrs. Davis behavior during the operation of her breast being cut out." Letter to Charles Wesley, 1 July 1758. Early Methodist Volume (EMV) 48, Methodist Archives and Research Centre (MARC). Quoted in Phyllis Mack, "Religious Dissenters in Enlightenment England," *History Workshop Journal* 49 (2000): 10.

2. The book focuses on "early English Methodism," understood as the Methodist movement in eighteenth-century England. Occasionally I extend this focus to developments that occurred in the movement during the early nineteenth century, such as the growth of Methodist support for the abolition of slavery.

3. General works on the meanings given to pain in different cultures include David B. Morris, *The Culture of Pain* (Berkeley and Los Angeles: University of California Press, 1991); Elaine Scarry, *The Body in Pain: The Making and Unmaking of the World* (Oxford: Oxford University Press, 1985).

4. Joseph Amato, *Victims and Values: A History and Theory of Suffering* (New York: Greenwood Press, 1990), 16.

5. Roy Porter, "Pain and Suffering," in *Companion Encyclopedia of the History of Medicine*, ed. W. F. Bynum and Roy Porter (London: Routledge, 1993), 2: 1575.

6. Amato, *Victims and Values*, 16.

7. Scarry, *The Body in Pain*, 4.

8. Morris, *The Culture of Pain*, 45. For a good recent discussion of the development of a "cultural history of pain," see Martha Stoddard Holmes and Tod Chambers, "Thinking through Pain," *Literature and Medicine* 24, no. 1 (2005): 127–41.

9. William M. Reddy, "Against Constructionism: The Historical Ethnography of Emotions," *Current Anthropology* 38, no. 3 (Jun., 1997): 329. Reddy provides a trenchant and useful critique of constructionism. He fails, however, to distinguish meaningfully between the "hard" constructionism that he criticizes and the more common "soft" constructionism that historians of emotion have tended to adopt. The latter assumes that there is a common human experience of emotion, but that the experience and expression of this is partially dependent on cultural context.

10. D. Bruce Hindmarsh, *The Evangelical Conversion Narrative: Spiritual Autobiography in Early Modern England* (New York: Oxford University Press, 2005), 158.

11. E. P. Thompson, *The Making of the English Working Class*, new ed. (London: Penguin Books, 1980), 409.

12. For Thompson's discussion of Wesleyan hymnody and its "masochistic" quality, see *The Making of the English Working Class*, 407–11. Thompson also briefly analyzes this tendency in Moravian hymns. For a response to Thompson, see David Hempton and John Walsh, "E. P. Thompson and Methodism," in *God and Mammon: Protestants, Money, and the Market, 1790–1860*, ed. Mark A. Noll (Oxford: Oxford University Press, 2002), 99–122.

13. Older biographies include Thomas Jackson, *The Life of the Rev. Charles Wesley*, 2 vols. (1841) and John Telford, *The Life of the Rev. Charles Wesley, M.A.* (London: Wesleyan-Methodist Book Room, 1900). More recent examples include Frederick C. Gill, *Charles Wesley: The First Methodist* (London: Lutterworth Press, 1964); T. Crichton Mitchell, *Charles Wesley: Man with the Dancing Heart* (Kansas City, Mo.: Beacon Hill, 1994); John R. Tyson, *Assist Me to Proclaim: The Life and Hymns of Charles Wesley* (Grand Rapids: Eerdmans, 2008).

14. Gareth Lloyd, *Charles Wesley and the Struggle for Methodist Identity* (Oxford: Oxford University Press, 2007).

15. Major works include J. Ernest Rattenbury, *The Evangelical Doctrines of Charles Wesley's Hymns* (London: Epworth, 1941); S. T. Kimbrough Jr., *Lost in Wonder: Charles Wesley, The Meaning of His Hymns Today* (Nashville: The Upper Room, 1987); John R. Tyson, *Charles Wesley on Sanctification: A Biographical and Theological Study* (Grand Rapids: Francis Asbury Press, 1986); Teresa Berger, *Theology in Hymns?* Trans. Timothy E. Kimbrough (Nashville: Kingswood Books, 1995). For a number of more recent theological studies, see Kenneth G. C. Newport and Ted A. Campbell, eds., *Charles Wesley: Life, Literature and Legacy* (Peterborough: Epworth, 2007).

16. Frank Baker produced several seminal works on Charles Wesley's hymns, including *Charles Wesley's Verse: An Introduction*, Second ed. (London: Epworth, 1988). See also J. R. Watson, "The Hymns of Charles Wesley and the Poetic Tradition," in *Charles Wesley: Life, Literature and Legacy*, 361–78; Donald Davie, *The Eighteenth-Century Hymn in England* (Cambridge: Cambridge University Press, 1993); Madeleine Forell Marshall and Janet Todd, *English Congregational Hymns in the Eighteenth Century* (Lexington: University Press of Kentucky, 1982).

17. Jeremy Gregory, "Charles Wesley and the Eighteenth Century," in *Charles Wesley: Life, Literature and Legacy*, 18–39.

Chapter One

Revisiting Charles Wesley

Prophet of ills why should I live,
Or by my sad forebodings grieve
Whom I can serve no more?
I only can their loss bewail
Till life's exhausted sorrows fail,
And the last pang is o'er.

Here then I quietly resign
Into those gracious hands Divine,
Whom I received from Thee,
My brethren and companions dear,
And finish with a parting tear
My useless ministry.[1]
Written After the Conference in Aug. 1780

At the age of seventy-three, Charles Wesley summarized his life and work in these gloomy terms. While this one poem, written in frustration, should not be taken as an entirely accurate portrayal of Wesley's self-perception, it does capture a recurring theme of melancholy and pain within both his life and his writings. Wesley's abiding fascination with suffering cannot be understood without reference to his own life and personality. As the following brief overview of his life and poetical work shows, many of his hymns were written in the midst of experiences of physical, emotional and spiritual hardship.

The Life of Charles Wesley

Charles Wesley was born in 1707, probably on 18 December, in the rectory at Epworth in Lincolnshire. His parents, Samuel and Susanna Wesley, had eighteen or nineteen children, of whom Charles was probably fifteenth or sixteenth. Much has been written about life in the Epworth rectory, and much of it is clouded in Methodist mythology.[2] Even apart from unverifiable anecdotes the household presents a distractingly dramatic story for biographers: the powerful personalities and marital battles of Susanna and Samuel; the imprisonment of Samuel for debt; the family's narrow escapes from death during the destruction of the rectory through fire; the visits of "Old Jeffrey," a poltergeist with a dislike for King William; and the various, occasionally scandalous, but generally miserable fates of the seven Wesley daughters. The most reliable sources about this period are the writings of Susanna Wesley and her children, which present obvious problems in interpretation. In addition, the centrality of John Wesley to Methodism means that far more material written to, by or about him, rather than Charles, has been retained. What sources we have present the picture of a family characterized by rigorous discipline of behavior, an intense piety, a strong emphasis on education, almost continual financial hardship and extremes of emotion in both affection and conflict.

From Susanna's explanation of her rather daunting child-rearing regime, it is clear that, like his brothers and sisters, Charles was taught from the age of one to "fear the rod and cry softly," learned his alphabet and could read by the age of five, was encouraged with praise and affirmation and was kept from contact with the local children as much as possible.[3] In all of this, the subjection of the will was paramount although, as is not always recognized, Susanna strongly emphasized the place of affection and positive reinforcement in child-rearing. In later years, Charles would affirm some of her principles in his own parenting.[4]

Historians have paid considerable attention to Susanna Wesley, both in her role as confidante and advisor to John (providing plenty of scope for oedipal theories), and more recently as an intellectual figure in her own right.[5] Her influence on Charles should be taken seriously, as they were close until her death in 1742.[6] Most historians of the Wesley family argue, however, that while John took after his mother, Charles was strikingly like his father.[7] While such a distinction relies too heavily on a depiction of Susanna as emotionally cool and controlled – a depiction that her writings fail to support – it does point to the fairly obvious parallels between Charles and his father. Samuel was Oxford-educated, a scholar by inclination and a poet. He wrote a *Life of Christ* in verse and his life's work was a lengthy commentary on Job. More similarities can be seen in Susanna's account of the conflict with Samuel that her political opinions provoked:

> 'Tis but a little while since he one evening observed in our family prayers I did not say amen to his prayer for K[ing] W[illiam] as I normally do to all others; upon which he retired to his study, and calling me to him asked me the reason of my not saying amen to the prayer. I was a little surprised at the question and don't well know what I answered, but too too well I remember what followed: He immediately kneeled down and imprecated the divine vengeance upon himself and all his posterity if ever he touched me more or came into a bed with me before I had begged God's pardon and his for not saying amen to the prayer for the K[ing].[8]

The explosive melodrama of this response (which resulted in a six-month separation) is highly reminiscent of Charles in situations of conflict later in life.

In 1716, Charles entered Westminster School and remained a student there until 1726. Throughout this period he lived with his oldest brother, Samuel, who was a schoolmaster at Westminster, and whose role in Charles's development has not been extensively explored. It is noteworthy that Charles lived with his brother throughout his adolescent years, and there are few records of his visiting home during this time. In describing his early life, Charles emphasized Samuel's importance to the family as a whole: "my eldest brother Samuel brought us up, and was a Father to the whole family."[9] Perhaps more significantly, Charles credited his brother with instilling in him the strict Churchmanship that would later bring him into so much conflict with other Methodists.[10] Samuel died suddenly in 1739, within several years of both Charles's parents.

From 1727 to 1735, Charles followed his brothers and father to Oxford, where he studied at Christ Church. After straying somewhat from the high ideals of his family, Charles became more consciously "serious" in his religious convictions and efforts and founded the small study group that became known to its detractors as "the Holy Club."[11] In his old age he recalled,

> My first year in College I lost in diversions. The next I set myself to study. Diligence led me into serious thinking. I went to the weekly sacrament, and persuaded 2 or 3 young scholars to accompany me, and to observe the method of study prescribed by the statutes of the University. This gained me the harmless nickname of Methodist. In half a year my brother left his curacy at Epworth, and came to our assistance. We then proceeded regularly in our studies, and in doing what good we could.[12]

This group has understandably been seen as an early model for Methodist societies, but it was hardly radical in either theology or behavior, and probably exactly suited Charles's high church principles.[13] The more significant change during this period was the extent to which Charles began to look to the leadership of his brother John. Some biographers have argued that Charles was influenced throughout his life by stronger personalities, that until this point he had deferred to his brother Samuel, but that from his Oxford days until his marriage he was under the sway of John.[14] Certainly, contemporaries noticed the enormous influence that John had on him. A member of the Holy Club claimed: "I never observed any person have a more real deference for another, than he constantly had for his brother... He followed his brother entirely. Could I describe one of them, I should describe both."[15]

John's influence was dramatically demonstrated in 1735, when he decided on a missionary venture to America. Charles was highly reluctant:

> I took my Master's Degree, and only thought of spending all my days at Oxford. But my brother, who had always the ascendant over me, persuaded me to accompany him and Mr Oglethorpe to Georgia. I exceedingly dreaded entering into holy orders; but he overruled me here also, and I was ordained Deacon... and the next Sunday, Priest.[16]

The time in Georgia was disastrous. He arrived in the midst of deep depression, convinced of his unworthiness for the task, writing to friends: "In vain have I fled from myself to America; I still groan under the intolerable weight of inherent misery!... Go where I will, I carry my hell about me."[17] Charles was soon estranged from Oglethorpe, whom he was assisting as secretary. He was deeply unpopular as a priest and became seriously ill very shortly after his arrival. The servants refused to wash his linen and his bed was removed from under him in the midst of his sickness. On 5 April 1736, less than a month after his arrival, a typical entry in his journal reads:

> At one this morning the sandflies forced me to rise, and smoke them out of the hut. The whole town was employed in the same manner. My congregation in the evening consisted of two Presbyterians and a Papist. I went home in great pain, my distemper being much increased with the little duty I could discharge.[18]

By the end of July Charles had resigned from his position and left Savannah. He was back in England by December. In his parting interview with Oglethorpe, with whom he had reconciled, the general recommended that Charles get married: "You are of a social temper, and would find in a married state the difficulties of working out your salvation exceedingly lessened."[19] Oglethorpe seems to have accurately identified Charles's desire for intimate relationships, a desire seen throughout Charles's life in the intensity of the relationships he formed, his delight in Methodist fellowship and the agonized hymns he composed on the loss of friends through death or discord.[20]

For both Wesley brothers, the brief sojourn in America seems to have been significant in simultaneously bringing them to a personal crisis point and introducing them to the Moravian spirituality that offered a solution to this crisis. The Moravians were European pietists, the remnants of a movement created by the proto-Protestant reformer Jan Huss. They were revitalized under the leadership of Count Nikolaus von Zinzendorf, who promoted the doctrine of salvation by faith alone, the experience of individual conversion or "new birth" and an intensely personal devotion to Jesus. In the first half of the eighteenth century, Moravians traveled to England and America to form missionary communities.[21] The Wesleys encountered Moravian missionaries en route to America, and on their return to England were introduced to the Moravian communities there.[22] The Moravians attempted to convince the brothers that their efforts towards salvation were in vain without the God-given experience of the "new birth."

From the time of his return to England until his conversion experience in May 1738, Charles's journal records repeated illness, great emotional upheaval and intense debates with Moravian pastors and lay people about the doctrines of justification by faith and personal assurance. He was deeply influenced during this period by the writings of both Zinzendorf and the Anglican nonjuror William Law.[23] Both men, working from quite different theological perspectives, stressed the importance of an inner religion and holiness in which Charles considered himself to be desperately lacking. An emphasis on true holiness – and a painful sense of sin – would remain significant throughout Charles's life, and form the theme of many of his hymns.

Having come to believe in the doctrine of justification by faith and the necessity of the new birth, Charles experienced conversion on 21 May 1738. Lying seriously ill and deeply distressed at the home of a Moravian brazier, he heard a woman's voice: "In the Name of Jesus of Nazareth arise and believe, and thou shalt be healed of all thy infirmities."[24] Believing that Christ had spoken to him (he was later told by the brazier's sister that she had been inspired by a dream to speak these words), he felt finally able to say that he did believe. In his description of the experience, which coincided with the beginning of his recovery, he emphasized the emotional peace his new convictions brought him.

> I now found myself at peace with God, and rejoiced in hope of loving Christ. My temper for the rest of the day was, mistrust of my own great, but before unknown weakness. I saw that by faith I stood; but by the continual support of faith, which kept me from falling, though of my own self I am ever sinking into sin. I went to bed sensible of my own weakness, (I humbly hope to be more and more so), yet content of Christ's protection.[25]

In outward terms, the experience of conversion resulted in a dramatic change of lifestyle for Charles. Central to his new convictions was the idea that this conversion experience, and the salvation it signified, should be offered to all. Following the example of his friend George Whitefield, and facing increasing opposition from local clergy in whose churches he attempted to preach, he took up field preaching.[26] For the next ten years, as an itinerant preacher, he preached up to five times a day, often to crowds of thousands.[27] As well, he administered the sacraments, counseled individuals, visited prisoners and attended deathbeds. His journal describes the physical attacks that he regularly faced during this time, as well as repeated bouts of serious sickness and depression.[28]

This early period of Charles's itinerancy is significant in marking the beginning of his regular production of poetic works, which were published by John from 1739 onwards. It was a period of intense upheaval within the revival, as the Wesleys parted ways with first the Moravians and then the Calvinist evangelicals. Charles was active in these controversies, writing polemical hymns, preaching sermons and arguing with individuals.

In 1747 Charles was introduced to Sarah ("Sally") Gwynne, nineteen years his junior and the daughter of a wealthy Welsh Methodist landowner. His attraction to her was apparently immediate, and his correspondence with her over the next two years shows the extremes of emotion that the prospect of marriage produced in him:

> Yet why should my complaints trouble one, whom I love and esteem infinitely more than ever? But my friendship is nothing worth "O wretched man that I am". How can I contribute to the happiness of another? I do not expect it: neither let those that love me; but rather fly from the reach of my sufferings.[29]

Charles and Sally were married on 8 April 1749. From all existing evidence the marriage was happy, and their voluminous correspondence provides the most extensive record of Charles's activities over the following forty years. After continuing his itinerant ministry for several years, Charles spent increasingly more time at home in Bristol with his family, and by 1756 was based firmly at home. He claimed that he was no longer well enough to travel continuously, but the Methodists were doubtful. "Matrimony has quite maimed poor Charles" was one verdict.[30]

In his early biography, John Telford concluded that Charles's depression and ill health was the result of his ceasing itinerant ministry: "There could have been no better tonic for him than that which his itinerant life supplied. He forgot himself in the joys of his glorious mission; when he ceased to travel he suffered and drooped."[31] Such an interpretation, with its implicit criticism of Wesley's retirement from the itinerancy, suited those for whom the heroic model of the itinerant preacher was beyond criticism. However, given the strains and trials of Wesley's experience of itinerancy (expressed to the point of desperation in his letters to Sally) it could equally be argued the trauma of these demanding years may have contributed to the illness and depression he experienced later in life.

Early biographers of Charles paid very little attention to his life and ministry after retirement from the itinerancy, though he remained an active leader of Methodism in Bristol and elsewhere.[32] John Whitehead's early biography, written in 1793, spends five pages of the two hundred and seventy-five discussing the thirty-three years of Charles's life after 1756. Only a couple of sentences refer to his ministry during this time.[33] This seems to reflect not only Methodist suspicion of Charles's zeal but the reluctance of Methodist biographers to discuss the personal and theological controversies in which Charles was embroiled during this period. Many of these controversies, particularly over the doctrine of perfection and the relationship between the Methodist movement and the Church of England, brought Charles into conflict with his brother John.

In these later years, Charles became increasingly disturbed about the possibility of Methodist separation from the Church of England. He was highly critical of the lay preachers, particularly their increasing agitation for permission to administer the sacraments. In several short hymns, he compared them to the biblical character Uzzah, who touched the ark of the covenant to prevent it from falling and was struck with leprosy.

> Behold your due to *Uzzah* dead
> For touching an external sign,
> You that the priestly right invade,
> And minister in things Divine!
> Will ignorance your bodies save?
> Inquire of *Uzzah* in his grave.[34]

These poetic denunciations were matched by furious battles with the lay preachers at the annual Methodist Conferences, by sermons exhorting the societies to stay within the Church and by continual politicking to gain support for his position among the supporters of Methodism.[35]

John's decision to ordain laymen in preparation for the Methodist work in America provoked further scathing poetic denunciations from Charles.

And is it come to this? and has the Man
On whose Integrity our Church relied,
Betray'd his trust, render'd our boastings vain,
And fal'n a Victim to ambitious Pride?[36]

At a less public level, John and Charles disagreed over the doctrine of perfection (the distinctive Methodist conviction that Christians could receive the ability to cease sinning) and over the place of suffering in the Christian life.

These doctrinal differences mirrored personal conflicts between the brothers. Perhaps the most famous was that caused by Charles's interference in John's marriage plans, just months after his own marriage. In September 1749, Charles received word that his brother was determined to marry Grace Murray, a Methodist follower. The reasons for his opposition to John's marriage are much debated and unclear, possibly centering on her involvement with another suitor, John Bennet, the potential negative impact of marriage on John's ministry or concerns about the lowly origins of Grace herself.[37] Whatever the case, Charles's reaction was immediate and frantic. Without informing John of his intentions, he rode from Bristol to Newcastle to find Grace and apparently collapsed at her feet, saying, "You have killed me."[38] He then virtually coerced her into marrying John Bennet and announced to John Wesley, "I renounce all intercourse with you, but what I would have with a heathen man or publican."[39]

While George Whitefield brought about some measure of reconciliation, this incident, along with Charles's marriage, marked the beginning of increasing personal tension between the brothers. John's letters exhorted Charles to further action and cooperation while Charles complained of being unappreciated and criticized his brother's decisions.[40] In 1766 John appealed to Charles:

> I think you and I have abundantly too little intercourse with each other. Are we not old acquaintances? Have we not known each other for half a century? And are we not jointly engaged in such a work as probably no two men upon earth are? Why then do we keep at such a distance? It is a mere device of Satan.[41]

It is difficult to gauge how serious the estrangement was – after both men had died, two of Charles's children argued the question, which suggests that even close family members were unable to judge.[42] Certainly the tension was more serious than many Methodist biographers have been willing to admit.[43] Gareth Lloyd has argued convincingly that Charles felt deeply and lastingly betrayed by John, and was unable to fully trust him ever again. Lloyd suggests that this personal grievance was a significant underlying emotional factor in Charles's passionate opposition to John's apparent encouragement of Methodist separation from the Church of England.[44]

Whether or not, as Brailsford and others argue, Sally replaced John as the directing influence in Charles's life, she certainly provided him with alternative companionship and emotional support throughout the latter part of his life. He grumbled when forced to spend time apart from his family: "They shall not get me here again in haste without my nurse and playfellows."[45] When Sally came to visit him in London, he urged her: "Bring my lovely boy and girl, if you have any bowels of compassion in you. 'Tis near nine weeks since I had a kiss from either of them."[46]

Charles and Sally had eight children. Five died in infancy and three – Samuel, Charles and Sarah – survived. Charles's letters and poems during this period record his emotional pain over the sicknesses and deaths of his children, his attempts to comfort Sally at the loss and his joy in the children that survived. After he received news of the death of one of their sons, Charles wrote to Sally:

> I received your trying news as of this morning; walked directly with my sympathising friend J- to take a place. All full, but the Bath-coach for tomorrow. I shall come thereby somewhat later to my beloved Sally and Charley and his sister. But the Lord is with you already; the Lord is with you always. This has been a solemn day. You must not deny my love to my sweet boy, if I am enabled to resign him for his heavenly Father to dispose of.[47]

Charles's own illnesses and depression continued and Sally survived smallpox in 1754.

Charles attempted to instill in his own children a valuing of discipline, piety and education similar to his own. By his own standards, he was only partially successful. From the first his two sons showed precocious musical ability, and Charles attempted to walk a fine line between developing their talent and offending Methodist sensibilities about performance. His cultivation of musical connections provoked Methodist ire. A friend warned him: "You have your enemies as well as your brother. They complain of your love for music, company and fine clothes, great folks and the want of your former zeal and frugality."[48] In 1769, Charles wrote a statement to be read at the Methodist society in Bristol, defending his decision to allow his son Charles to play music for profit. Charles argued for allowing his son to do the work to which his talents led him:

> We do not enough attend to the natural bent and turn of our children, in settling them to this or that particular way of life; which occasions the miscarriage of so many. What numbers have been ruined by being forced to unsuitable trades and professions![49]

Music was a respectable trade, Charles argued: God had "been pleased to make good use of vocal music among us. Our hymns have helped to spread the Gospel: God himself has owned, and applied them to many of your hearts."[50]

Charles's second son, Samuel, became a famous organist and composer, but rebelled against the strictures of Methodism. He temporarily converted to Roman Catholicism, an act that resulted in some of Charles's most personally anguished poems. Samuel's letters, many of them written to his sister after their father's death, are a useful but neglected source of information about the family life of the Wesleys. During Charles's life their relationship was strained, though in later life Samuel became increasingly positive towards his father's memory and composed music in honor of "his dictates."[51] The other two children, Sarah and Charles, were more conformist, remaining loyal to their father, though not necessarily to Methodism. Charles's letters to them suggest deep affection struggling against an awkward formality. He wrote plaintively to his daughter:

> I think you may avail yourself of my small knowledge of books and poetry. I am not yet too old to assist you a little in your reading, and perhaps improve your taste in versifying. You need not dread my severity. I have a laudable partiality for my own children. Witness your brothers, whom I do not love a jot better than you; only be as ready to show me your verses as they their music.[52]

After a long decline, Charles Wesley died on 29 March 1788. Accounts of his death emphasized that he fulfilled Methodist expectations of a "good" death: praying for his enemies, affirming his faith in God and exhorting his children.[53] Several days before his death, he dictated a final poem to his wife:

> In age and feebleness extreme,
> Who shall a helpless worm redeem?
> Jesus! my only hope Thou art,
> Strength of my failing flesh and heart;
> Oh! could I catch one smile from Thee
> And drop into eternity![54]

By his own request, he was buried in the consecrated ground of the graveyard of St Mary-le-bone, the parish church he had attended while living in London.

The Writings of Charles Wesley

Though Charles Wesley's reputation suffered somewhat at the hands of early Methodist historians, he left an extensive body of published and unpublished writings for historians to make use of. His writings can be divided into four broad categories: poetical works, letters, journal and sermons. His poetical works, which will be examined in more detail in the following chapter, remain his most famous achievement. Latest estimates suggest he wrote about 9,000 hymns or poems, most of which were composed after his conversion experience in 1738.[55] He wrote on a wide variety of subjects, primarily spiritual and theological, but also more "secular," though he would have been unlikely to recognize the validity of such a distinction. He wrote hymns for the unsaved and for the new believer, for those rejoicing and those mourning, for the condemned criminal, the sick and for children. He wrote more doctrinally instructive hymns on themes such as the trinity or the sacraments. Often such hymns were distinctly polemical, addressing specific issues in controversies with the Calvinists, Moravians and others. Charles's domestic life also inspired hundreds of poems, from the anguish and hope of his courtship poems, to the whimsical rhymes he wrote for his young children to the outpourings of despair in his poems about his son Samuel. In later life he also wrote poems on political issues such as the American War of Independence and the Gordon Riots, displaying his political conservatism, intense loyalty to the King and dislike of "the Mob."

Letter-writing played a significant role in fostering co-operation and sharing news among those involved in the evangelical revivals that took place across Europe and America in the eighteenth century.[56] The Wesleys wrote to an extensive circle of followers, friends and fellow-revivalists. They were bombarded with letters from Methodists seeking advice and reassurance and wrote to many in return.[57] Around 650 letters written by Charles Wesley are extant, providing valuable insights into his life and character.[58] Many of these letters were written to his wife Sally during his absences on preaching trips. They contain details of his daily activities, news about the societies and regular descriptions of his state of health. Letters to fellow Methodist preachers reveal information about his involvement in theological and political or personal clashes within the movement. Most of these letters are pastoral rather than doctrinal, with a few significant exceptions that give insights into his theological views on topics such as eschatology.[59]

Charles's journal has provided the main primary material utilized by biographers. He may well have begun writing a daily journal during his years at Oxford, when he wrote to John: "I would willingly write a diary of my actions, but don't know how to go about it... I'm fully convinced of the usefulness of such an undertaking."[60] The extant portion of his diary begins with his arrival in Georgia in 1736 and continues, at times sketchily, only until 1756. A large proportion of this was published by Thomas Jackson, one of Charles's earliest biographers, and this published version remains the one that most biographers use. The journal is primarily a record of his itinerant years and as such gives insight into the drama and conflict of those years, as seen through Charles's perception of the meaning of Methodism and his own place in it. Unfortunately, Jackson edited the original journal, leaving out sections in shorthand or which he considered unedifying.[61] The original manuscript of the journal is currently in the process of being decoded and published in a complete edition. It certainly has more to reveal about Charles's inner life.[62]

Finally, between thirteen and twenty-three sermons of Charles Wesley's are extant.[63] The number is uncertain because authorship is not always clear, given the Wesleys' tendency to preach each other's sermons. The recent identification and publication of these sermons sheds light upon the neglected question of Charles as Methodist preacher, the role in which he spent so much of his life. One of his sermons, "Awake Thou That Sleepest," first preached before the University of Oxford, became the most frequently published Methodist tract of the Wesleys' lifetime. Others, such as "On the Cause and Cure of Earthquakes," give rare prose examples of Charles's extended theological reasoning.

Together, these writings provide a rich source of material for interpreting Charles Wesley's life and thought. They illuminate the Methodist culture that he helped to form. They also provide some important personal context for the strong and undoubtedly unusual emphasis on suffering within his hymns.

Charles Wesley and Suffering

In spite of the wealth of sources available to the historian, there is no simple answer to the question of why Charles Wesley became so concerned with the experience of overwhelming pain. His experiences, temperament and theological formation all appear to have played a part in this development. The hardships of his own life were certainly significant: a tumultuous childhood, lifelong ill health, years of physically and emotionally demanding itinerant ministry, serious conflicts with his brother John, the early deaths of five of his children, his son Samuel's emotional instability and conversion to Roman Catholicism and the (to Charles) heartbreaking movement of Methodism away from the Church of England. Some of these events, such as the upheavals of his childhood, were (as far as we know) left unmentioned in his writings or, in the case of the persecution he experienced, identified as experiences of suffering that he was able to overcome. This does not mean that they left him untouched. Other experiences Charles explicitly lamented in both hymns and prose. From these writings, it seems that the conflict with his brother over John's brief engagement and eventual marriage, the move of Methodism away from the established Church and the experiences of bereavement and estrangement within his own family were particularly painful. That these experiences occurred later in Charles's life help explain the growing emphasis on suffering within his hymns during this period.

These painful events combined with (and surely contributed to) a tendency towards what would in modern terms be called depression. Though he clearly knew times of joy, peace and satisfaction, Charles's personal writings make constant reference to distressing emotional struggles from early on in his life. This was not simply the sense of unworthiness and fear of judgment that preceded his evangelical conversion. His letters from America, written before conversion, and his letters to Sally, written well after his conversion, both speak of regular experiences of deep emotional distress, which seem to have arisen from a deep sense of weakness and inability that at times overwhelmed him. In the language of his time, he would probably have been understood as prone to "melancholy."[64]

Charles also interpreted his experiences in the context of a theological tradition that had much to say about suffering. His early exposure to the writings of theologians like Thomas a Kempis and William Law, with their heavy emphasis on the importance of self-denial and the value of suffering, provided him with an interpretive framework for understanding the hardships he experienced and observed.[65] As will be discussed in the following chapter, his own brother thought that it was this early doctrinal influence that was responsible for his emphasis on suffering.

Charles Wesley's experiences, personality and theological formation do not provide a simple explanation for the theme of overwhelming pain that emerges in his poetical works. They do, however, help to provide a context for interpreting that theme, particularly its increasing emphasis within his poetical works in later life, as well as his conclusion that his life was one of "exhausted sorrows" and his ministry had been "useless."

Notes

1. "Written After the Conference in Aug. 1780, The Last Which the Writer Was Present At." [unpublished] *PW* 8: 416.

2. Biographies of Charles that include details about his childhood are cited throughout this chapter. Henry Rack describes the Wesley brothers' childhood (with emphasis on John's experience) in *Reasonable Enthusiast: John Wesley and the Rise of Methodism*, Third ed. (London: Epworth Press, 2002), 45–60. Two recent studies of Charles Wesley that include extensive biographical material are Tyson, *Assist Me To Proclaim* and Lloyd, *Charles Wesley and the Struggle for Methodist Identity*.

3. Susanna Wesley to John Wesley, 25 Oct. 1732, in Charles Wallace, ed., *Susanna Wesley* (Oxford, New York: Oxford University Press, 1997), 369–73.

4. See Charles Wesley to Sally Wesley, 16 Aug. 1766. DDCW 7/88.

5. A recent scholarly biography that places Susanna more firmly in theological and historical context is John A. Newton, *Susanna Wesley and the Puritan Tradition in Methodism* (London: Epworth Press, 2002). Charles Wallace provides analysis and commentary in his introductions to the material in Wallace, ed., *Susanna Wesley*.

6. The preserved letters written by Susanna to Charles suggest that Charles did not correspond with his mother as often as John did before the death of their father, but that Charles became closer to his mother after her husband and oldest son died. In early 1739 she wrote to him, "You cannot more desire to see me than I do to see you... I am in a state of great temptation and want to talk with you about many things. I need your direction and instruction how to act in the present situation..." Susanna Wesley to Charles Wesley, 27 Dec. 1739. Wallace, ed., *Susanna Wesley*, 180.

7. Rack, *Reasonable Enthusiast*, 51.

8. Susanna Wesley to Lady Yarborough, 7 Mar. 1702. Wallace, ed., *Susanna Wesley*, 35.

9. Charles Wesley to John Langshaw, 17 May 1779. Arthur W. Wainwright, ed., *Wesley-Langshaw Correspondence: Charles Wesley, His Sons and the Lancaster Organists* (Emory: Scholars Press, 1993), 34.

10. Charles Wesley to Dr. Chandler, 28 Apr. 1785. DDWES 1/38.

11. One of the few letters from Charles's early days at Oxford shows him describing a failed romance with an actress whom he describes as "a Whore." Charles Wesley to John Wesley, 5–22 Jan. 1729. DDCW 1/2.

12. Wesley to Chandler, DDWES 1/38.

13. Kenneth Newport, ed., *The Sermons of Charles Wesley: A Critical Edition with Introduction and Notes* (Oxford: Oxford University Press, 2001), 14.

14. Mabel Richmond Brailsford, *A Tale of Two Brothers: John and Charles Wesley* (London: Rupert Hart-Davies, 1954), 60–61, 231. Gareth Lloyd supports aspects of Brailsford's interpretation in *Charles Wesley and the Struggle for Methodist Identity*.

15. John Gambold quoted by Brailsford, *A Tale of Two Brothers*, 74.

16. Wesley to Chandler, DDWES 1/38.

17. Charles Wesley to Sally Kirkham and Anne Granville, 5, 14 Feb. 1736. DDCW 1/6.

18. 5 April 1736. *CWJ* 1: 16.

19. 25 July 1736. *CWJ* 1: 35.

20. For example, *HSP* (1739): "Upon Parting With His Friends (Parts I–V)." *PW* 1: 244–49.

21. For an account of the Moravian presence in England during this period, see Colin Podmore, *The Moravian Church in England, 1728–1760* (Oxford: Clarendon Press, 1995).

22. Rack gives a detailed account of John Wesley's contact with the Moravians both during and after his trip to America, with some reference to Charles. Rack, *Reasonable Enthusiast*, 121–23, 37–45. Telford describes Charles's meetings with Zinzendorf and the Moravian missionary Peter Bohler. Telford, *The Life of the Rev. Charles Wesley, M.A.*, 59, 67–71.

23. Gill, *Charles Wesley*, 65. William Law had been a significant influence on the Wesleys well before this point.

24. 21 May 1738. *CWJ* 1: 90.

25. 21 May 1738. *CWJ* 1: 92.

26. 24 June 1739. *CWJ* 1: 155.

27. Telford, *The Life of the Rev. Charles Wesley, M.A.*, 124.

28. For examples of sickness, depression and persecution, see 15–18 March 1740, *CWJ* 1: 195–200; 29 July–7 Sept. 1740, *CWJ* 1: 247–48; 25–29 May 1743, *CWJ* 1: 309–10; 31 Aug. 1743, *CWJ* 1: 331; 16 Sept. 1746, *CWJ* 1: 428; 21–26 Feb. 1747, *CWJ* 1: 442–44; 20 Oct. 1748, *CWJ* 2: 42; 1 Dec. 1749, *CWJ* 2: 66.

29. Charles Wesley to Sally Gwynne, 12 Mar. 1749. DDCW 5/38.

30. Comment by John Berridge, who added that Whitefield and John Wesley's wives were "a brace of ferrets." Rack, *Reasonable Enthusiast*, 255.

31. Telford, *The Life of the Rev. Charles Wesley, M.A.*, 308.

32. Gareth Lloyd, "Charles Wesley and His Biographers: An Exercise in Methodist Hagiography," *Bulletin of the John Rylands University Library of Manchester* 82, no. 1 (2000): 83.

33. Lloyd, "Charles Wesley and His Biographers," 83.

34. *SHSPHS* (1762): "2 Sam. 6: 7." *PW* 9: 165.

35. For a thorough discussion of Charles's conflict with the preachers, based on primary sources, see Lloyd, *Charles Wesley and the Struggle for Methodist Identity*, 110–211.

36. *Ordination Hymns*: "Occidit! Occidit!" *UP* 3: 87.

37. Charles's diary suggests that his primary concern with John getting married may have been that John had publicly recommended celibacy for the clergy and so would be seen as hypocritical. Charles's (shorthand) entry for 3 June 1750 reads, "Weighed down all day by my brother's threat to marry. O why did he ever prelude himself from it? Why did he publish his rash book against it?" (Ken Newport's translation).

38. Brailsford, *A Tale of Two Brothers*, 200.

39. Newport, ed., *Sermons*, 23.

40. See Gareth Lloyd, "Charles Wesley: A New Evaluation of His Life and Ministry" (PhD diss., University of Liverpool, 2002), 180–85.

41. John Wesley to Charles Wesley, 27 June 1766. John Wesley, *The Works of John Wesley*, 14 vols., vol. 12 (Grand Rapids: Zondervan, 1958), 130.

42. See the exchange of letters between Samuel III and Sarah Wesley Jr., published in Michael Kassler and Philip Olleson, eds., *Samuel Wesley (1766–1837): A Source Book* (Aldershot: Ashgate, 2001), 142–43.

43. For example, Telford, *The Life of the Rev. Charles Wesley, M.A.*, 195.

44. Lloyd, *Charles Wesley and the Struggle for Methodist Identity*, 88–133.

45. Charles Wesley to Sarah Wesley, 9 Sept. 1764. *CWJ* 2: 229.

46. Charles Wesley to Sally Wesley, 3 July [1763]. DDCW 7/90.

47. Charles Wesley to Sally Wesley, nd. DDCW 7/14. It is not clear to which son this letter refers.

48. John Fletcher to Charles Wesley, quoted in D. M. Jones, *Charles Wesley: A Study* (London: Skeffington, 1919), 235.

49. Charles Wesley, "Intended to be read in the society at Bristol," Feb. 1769. DDWES 4/83.

50. Wesley, "Intended to be read in the society at Bristol."

51. Samuel Wesley III to Vincent Novello. Kassler and Olleson, eds., *Samuel Wesley*, 397.

52. Charles Wesley to Sarah Wesley Jr., 11 Oct. 1777. John R Tyson, ed., *Charles Wesley: A Reader* (New York: Oxford University Press, 1989), 353–54.

53. Sally described Charles's death in a letter to John Wesley, 4 Apr. 1788. Tyson, ed., *Charles Wesley*, 482.

54. "Lines Dictated on His Death Bed." Tyson, ed., *Charles Wesley*, 481.

55. Newport, ed., *Sermons*, 4f.

56. W. R. Ward, *The Protestant Evangelical Awakening* (Cambridge: Cambridge University Press, 1992), 2. See also Susan O'Brien, "A Transatlantic Community of Saints: The Great Awakening and the First Evangelical Network, 1735–1755," *American Historical Review* 91, no. 4 (1986): 811–32.

57. Hundreds of letters to John and Charles are preserved in the Early Methodist Volumes in the Methodist Archives and Research Centre at the John Rylands University Library (JRULM).

58. The MARC holds by far the largest collection of letters written by Charles Wesley. Around 600 are contained in the Charles Wesley and Wesley Family collections.

59. Tyson, ed., *Charles Wesley*, 13. There are notable exceptions to this, for example Charles's lengthy exploration of eschatology in a letter written in 1754. This has been discussed in detail by Kenneth Newport, "Charles Wesley's Interpretation of Some Biblical Prophecies according to a Previously Unpublished Letter Dated 25 April 1754," *Bulletin of the John Rylands University Library of Manchester* 77 (1995): 31–52.

60. Tyson, ed., *Charles Wesley*, 10.

61. Newport, ed., *Sermons*, 8.

62. Kenneth Newport, who is undertaking this process, has very kindly given me access to the portions that he has transcribed so far.

63. See Newport, ed., *Sermons*.

64. The understanding of "melancholy" as a medical problem considerably pre-dated the eighteenth century, but was understood during this period as a particularly English problem. The leading expert on melancholy and related nervous disorders during this time was the famous Dr. George Cheyne. See George Cheyne, *The English Malady: or, a treatise of nervous diseases of all kinds, as spleen, vapours, lowness of spirits, hypochondriacal and hysterical distempers* (London, 1733).

65. For a discussion of the influence of William Law and other High Church theologians on John and Charles's early thought, particularly with regards to suffering, see Geordan Hammond, "Restoring Primitive Christianity: John Wesley and Georgia, 1735–1737" (PhD diss., University of Manchester, 2008), 49–64.

Chapter Two

Revisiting the Hymns of Charles Wesley

In December 1788, six months after Charles's death, John Wesley dedicated a week to reading over a collection of his brother's unpublished verse. He recorded his verdict on the poems in his journal:

> Some are bad; some mean, some most excellently good: They give the true sense of Scripture, always in good English, generally in good verse; many of them are equal to most, if not to any, he ever wrote; but some still savour of that poisonous mysticism, with which we were both not a little tainted before we went to America. This gave a gloomy cast, first to his mind, and then to many of his verses: This made him frequently describe religion as a melancholy thing.[1]

As John noted, suffering – spiritual, emotional or physical – is a major theme of thousands of Charles Wesley's poetical works. Repeatedly, Charles reflected on the experience of those in overwhelming pain: the bleeding and thirsty Jesus, the believer feeling forsaken by God, the woman racked with the agony of childbirth, the parent grieving over a child's rebellion. For John, who earlier in 1788 had commented on "having had so little pain in my life; and so little sorrow, or anxious care,"[2] such reflections were unnecessarily gloomy and theologically suspect. His verdict on Charles's hymns obscures, however, the extent to which these works represent a determined and extensive engagement with the experience of suffering. For their eighteenth-century readers and singers, the hymns provided a powerful model for how Christians should experience, interpret and respond to suffering.

Analyzing the construction of suffering in Wesley's hymns requires an interpretive framework. How should Wesley's verse be read and understood? Answering this question requires attention to genre as much as to text: simply abstracting propositions about suffering from Wesley's verse and reconstructing them into a theological system could easily misrepresent his thinking. Equally, it is not enough to construct a standard definition for the genre of "hymn"; rather, Wesley's own use and development of the genre(s) in which he wrote must be considered. Literary genres, like all cultural forms, possess contexts and histories.[3] Close attention must therefore be paid to the personal and cultural context in which Wesley wrote, to his own understanding and experience of hymn-singing, as well as to the relationship between the ideas expressed and the forms in which he expressed them. Revisiting, in this way, the question of how Wesley's hymns should be interpreted, will provide us with a new understanding of his significance within early Methodism as a whole.

The Hymns of Charles Wesley

The hymns generally attributed to Charles Wesley may be conveniently divided into three categories: those published prior to his engagement and marriage in 1749, those published between 1749 and his death and those that remained unpublished during his lifetime.[4] This division allows particular attention to be paid to questions of context, editing and authorship. From 1739 until 1749, the major collections in which Charles's verse appeared were edited by, and published in partnership with, his brother John. Following their conversion experiences during 1738, the brothers jointly published *Hymns and Sacred Poems* in 1739. This collection, the first of many with the same title, included translations and paraphrases of the work of other authors, as well as a number of original poems by the brothers. They then published another four collections of *Hymns and Sacred Poems* between 1740 and 1747. Charles's work was also published in his brother's three-volume *A Collection of Moral and Sacred Poems* in 1744.

All of these collections present the scholar with some difficulties, because in them the brothers chose not to indicate the individual authorship of the verses that were their own compositions. Charles was by far the more prolific poet, but both brothers wrote verse, making it difficult to argue that John was involved only in the work of translating or editing. Where there is no external reference (such as an original manuscript in Charles's handwriting) to determine who wrote a particular hymn, various scholars have suggested internal criteria for identifying the work of each brother.[5] These criteria are suggestive rather than conclusive, and most scholars agree that, while the vast majority is the work of Charles, it is ultimately impossible to be sure of the authorship of some of the early hymns.[6] As I will argue below, however, most of the hymns that focus on suffering can be attributed with some confidence to Charles.

During this same period, Charles also published a number of shorter collections under his own or his brother's name. The titles give some idea of the range of subject matter of his compositions. They include the anti-Calvinist *Hymns on God's Everlasting Love* in 1741, *Hymns for Times of Trouble and Persecution* in 1744, *Hymns for the Nativity of Our Lord* and *Hymns on the Lord's Supper* in 1745, and *Hymns to the Trinity*, *Funeral Hymns* and *Hymns for Children* in 1746. All these poems were written during the period of Charles's itinerancy and reflect the upheaval of those years, including the Calvinist controversy and the threats of Jacobite uprising that created so much suspicion of the Methodists. While it is difficult to know how much editorial involvement John had in these works, it may have been extensive, given Charles's deference to his brother during this period. When making later use of verses from these collections in Methodist hymnbooks, John edited them significantly. His criticisms and editorial choices with regard to these works and others provide valuable evidence of how the brothers differed in their theological views and support for the contention that those poems dealing primarily with the question of suffering are unlikely to have been the work of John. Both the subject matter and style of these works suggest that Charles composed them.

First, the interest in the individual's struggle with physical or emotional pain, displayed in many of these poems, suggests that they were written by Charles. As the quotation at the beginning of this chapter implies, John rejected the possibility that the religious life should be a "melancholy thing." His own description of his personality (which tallies with that of his closest observers) emphasized his even temper: "Almost ever since I can remember I have been led in a particular way. I go in an even line, being very little raised at one time or depressed at another."[7] While John's letters reflect more emotional turmoil than this self-evaluation would suggest, it is still difficult to identify him with the intense physical and emotional anguish that is described in so many of these poems.[8] Charles would go on to write poems of this intensely emotional nature throughout his life, while there is little evidence of John's doing so.[9]

In sermons, John preached against the idea (clearly contained in Charles's hymns) that suffering was of more benefit to the Christian than was joy.

> Is not the work of God in the heart most swiftly and effectually carried on during a state of inward suffering? Is not a believer more swiftly and thoroughly purified by sorrow than by joy? By anguish and pain and distress and spiritual martyrdoms than by continual peace? So the *mystics* teach; so it is written in their books – but not in the *oracles of God.* The Scripture nowhere says that the absence of God best perfects his work in the heart.... Joy in the Holy Ghost will far more effectually purify the soul than the want of that joy.[10]

John's argument echoes his complaint about the "poisonous mysticism" that had infected his brother. Here mysticism is understood as affirming the role of suffering to a degree that John found unscriptural, a criticism that he also leveled at Charles. The brothers' opinions about the role of suffering amounted to a significant and lifelong theological difference between them.

Second, John consistently criticized the emotive style of Charles's verse, a style particularly evident in his writing on suffering.[11] John disliked what he termed the "namby-pambical" tendency or the use of "fondling expression" in hymns.[12] From the pattern of his editorial decisions when re-publishing Charles's work, John seems to have been referring to such issues as physicality or sentimentality. He edited out words such as "kiss" or "sweet" in relation to Christ; detailed descriptions of the blood and wounds of Christ; and phrases such as "dear Lord" or "dear Saviour."[13] Discussing the use of the term "dear" with reference to Christ, John exhorted the Methodists:

> Do we not frequently use this unscriptural expression of our Lord in private conversation also? And are we not then especially apt to speak of him as a mere man? Particularly when we are describing his sufferings, how easily do we slide

> into this! We do well to be cautious in this matter. Here is not room for indulging a warm imagination. I have sometimes almost scrupled singing (even in the midst of my brother's excellent hymn)
>
> "That dear, disfigured face,"
>
> or that glowing expression,
>
> "Drop thy warm blood upon my heart,"
>
> lest it should seem to imply the forgetting I am speaking of "the man that is my fellow, saith the Lord of hosts."[14]

John's sermon "On Knowing Christ after the Flesh" demonstrates that his concern over the language in Charles's hymns stemmed particularly from a desire to distance himself from the Moravians, whose hymns he identified as full of "fondling expression."[15] While John's scruples seemed to relate particularly to a concern that appropriate reverence be shown for the divine person of Christ, they also suggest a discomfort with physicality and, combined with his concerns over Charles's "melancholy" understanding of religion, a lack of interest in extended reflection on the experience of suffering.[16] Therefore, in spite of the overarching questions of authorship and editorial control that are raised by John's involvement in the publication of Charles's early works, verses dealing primarily with suffering may with some confidence be cited or quoted as Charles's work.

In 1749, keen to prove his financial stability to his future parents-in-law, Charles published a double volume of *Hymns and Sacred Poems*. John was not involved in this publication. "In the year 1749," he recorded, "my brother printed two volumes of 'hymns and sacred poems'. As I did not see these before they were published, there were some things in them I did not approve of."[17] From this point on, Charles seems to have published most of his new verse without John's participation, and the latter part of his life proved the more fruitful in terms of poetical output. He attributed at least part of his productiveness to the deterioration of his health, commenting in the preface of one work that "God, having graciously laid His hand upon my body, and disabled me for the principal work of the ministry, has thereby given me an unexpected occasion of writing the following hymns."[18]

Charles's solo publications during this period included *Hymns and Spiritual Songs* in 1753, *An Epistle to the Reverend Mr. John Wesley* in 1755, *Hymns on the Expected Invasion* in 1759, the mammoth *Short Hymns on Select Passages of the Holy Scriptures* in 1762, *Hymns for the Use of Families* in 1767, *An Elegy on the late Reverend George Whitefield* in 1771 and *Prayers for Condemned Malefactors* in 1785. In addition, he supplied hymns that were published as appendages to John's polemical essays. In 1760, for example, the brothers published an essay entitled *Reasons against a Separation from the Church of England... With hymns for the preachers among the Methodists (so called).* Though composed by Charles, these hymns were presumably vetted by John. For the most part, however, poetical works published during this later period may be taken as Charles's unedited work. John continued to criticize his brother's verse. Commenting on *Short Hymns on Select Passages of the Holy Scriptures*, he wrote to a Methodist laywoman to "take care you are not hurt by anything in the 'short Hymns', contrary to the doctrines you have long received."[19]

At Charles's death, in 1788, about half of his verse seems to have been unpublished. The subject matter of some of this work suggests that it was kept private because of its personal nature. It includes jingles for his children, furious denunciations of the American rebels during the War of Independence, attacks on his brother John, and agonized outpourings of grief on occasions such as the conversion of his son Samuel to Roman Catholicism.[20] Also left unpublished was part of the *Short Hymns on Select Passages of Scripture*. While it is tempting to see all of this work as offering a particularly uncensored view of Wesley's opinions and emotions, his decision not to publish may equally reflect a dissatisfaction with what he had written. More importantly, the majority of these hymns were probably not sung or read by many others. While these hymns are important for a broad understanding of Wesley's thought, their impact on early Methodist culture was obviously limited.

Characteristics of Wesley's Hymns

The existing literary and historical scholarship on Charles Wesley's hymns contains a wide range of opinions on both the literary value and the literary characteristics of his verse. For our purposes, it is particularly significant that alternative understandings of the nature of Wesley's hymns produce alternative approaches to the ideas they contain. Some scholars have chosen to read the hymns as a straightforward representation of Wesley's innermost feelings, little different from a prose journal.[21] Others have argued that, on the contrary, congregational hymns such as Wesley wrote are characterized by their impersonality.[22] On such a reading, it is impossible to gain insight into Wesley's personal emotions and opinions from his hymns. From this assumption, literary scholars Marshall and Todd argue that the hymns represent "not the expressive *venting* of feeling but rather the evangelical *directing* of feeling."[23] The ideas about suffering that they contain express only "doctrinally corrected" responses to suffering. Given such divergent views of the basic nature of Wesley's verse, it is clearly necessary to explore further the nature and purpose of this verse in general before analyzing specific poems.

Wesley's work is characterized by variety. Even the brief survey of his work given above should discourage the tendency to treat all his verse as belonging to one easily defined genre. While many (though not all) of his poems were published in collections described as "hymns," his 9,000 works included verse identified by the author as belonging to a range of genres: elegies, epistles, epitaphs and "sacred poems." In addition, many of the works identified as hymns display quite different approaches to the genre. While considering marriage to Sally Gwynne, Wesley wrote a number of what he described as "Deliberating Hymns." One of these, included in a letter to Sally, illustrates their general tone. It begins:

1. And is there hope for me
In life's distracting maze,

And shall I live on earth to see
A few unruffled days?
A man of sorrow I,
A sufferer from the womb,
'Twas all my hope in peace to die,
And rest within my tomb.

2. How then can I conceive
A good for me designed,
The greatest God himself could give
The parent of mankind?
A good by sovereign love
To sinless Adam given
His joyous paradise t'improve,
And turn his earth to heaven.

3. God of unbounded grace,
If yet thou wilt bestow,
On me, the vilest of the race,
The choicest gift below;
My drooping heart prepare
The blessing to receive,
And bid the child of sad despair
With confidence believe.[24]

This "Deliberating Hymn" is entirely different in style and tone from other poems also described as hymns. For example, the collection of *Short Hymns on Select Passages of Scripture* includes a hymn on 1 Samuel 1: 23, a verse that reads "The woman gave her son suck, until she weaned him." In his hymn, Wesley uses this description of the prophet Samuel's mother to pass judgment on the mothers of eighteenth-century England.

Not like the mothers of our day,
Who of all care themselves divest,
And thrust their new-born babes away,
And hang them on another's breast.[25]

This brief comment on a social question of the day is included in a collection described as "hymns," but it seems to belong to an entirely different genre. This variety in style and tone within Wesley's work is easier to understand when seen within the context of the historical development of the genre of "hymn."

The eighteenth century witnessed the fierce continuation of an old debate about the place of songs in English congregational worship. The English reformers, following Calvin rather than Luther, minimized the role of music in worship. The 1559 Act of Uniformity permitted the use of a "modest distinct song" before or after the service of common prayer, but for 200 years this was interpreted restrictively to allow only paraphrased psalms.[26] Individuals occasionally published non-scriptural lyrics for use in personal devotion or for the lesser services of morning and evening prayer.[27] While hymn-singing became acceptable in some Nonconformist congregations during the seventeenth century (and leading Puritans such as Richard Baxter and John Bunyan wrote hymns) this served to associate hymns with theological and political radicalism.

In the late seventeenth and early eighteenth centuries, a debate raged over the question of hymn-singing in sermons, tracts, magazines and letters to the editor.[28] Were poetic lyrics (and music) an aid to devotion or a dangerous distraction? Would the introduction of extra-biblical lyrics smuggle human opinions into the divine service? Would they lead congregations toward the irrationality and emotionalism of Papacy and Nonconformism, or could they prove a vital weapon in the Church's competition with these forces? In this debate, hymns seem to have been broadly understood as songs for Christian worship with extra-biblical lyrics. Critics saw hymn-writing as part of a general decline toward irrationality and anti-authoritarianism. An irate reviewer of Charles Wesley's *Short Hymns on Select Passages of Scripture* exclaimed:

> Indeed the irreverent treatment which the bible continually meets with, IN THIS PROTESTANT COUNTRY, from the swarms of hackney commentators, expositors and enthusiastic hymn-makers, would almost provoke the rational Christian to applaud even the *Church of Rome* for the care she has taken to secure it from vulgar profanation.[29]

In spite of such criticisms, the number of hymns and hymnbooks published increased rapidly throughout the eighteenth century.[30] While these hymns were used mostly in association with the evangelical revivals, they were part of a wider trend of popular devotional music and poetry, including the sacred oratorios spearheaded by Handel, and devotional poems by writers such as Anne Steele. The eighteenth century saw the publication of collections such as Isaac Watts' *Hymns and Spiritual Songs*, the Wesley brothers' *Hymns and Sacred Poems* and the anonymous *The Sincere Christian's Devout Companion*. Each of these collections contains devotional poems or lyrics, capable of being set to music, published privately and sold to individuals. The distinction between "hymns," "spiritual songs" or "sacred poems" is nowhere in these works made clear. This all suggests that, at the time Wesley was writing, the genre of "hymn" was not rigidly defined: it was still an experimental and controversial genre.

If Wesley's work is characterized by diversity, it is also notable for the profound moral and spiritual significance that he gave to emotion. Literary scholar Donald Davie notes that, reading Wesley after the works of earlier hymn-writers such as Watts, one is struck by "a steep rise in the emotional temperature assumed or exacted of us as readers (or singers)."[31] Wesley's poetry often deals with Christian doctrines that he held to be objectively true: the triune nature of God, the incarnation, the atoning death of Christ and the resurrection of the dead. His writing is densely theological, compressing complex doctrine into pithy phrases such as "Beings Source begins to Be,/ And God Himself is Born!"[32] Yet the subjective response to these doctrines receives as much, if not more, attention from Wesley. A theological basis for this subjectivity is found in the Methodist emphasis on emotional or "sensible" experience.

Much has been written about the importance of experience in early Methodist theology, particularly within the thought of John Wesley.[33] John preached the necessity of faith and a new birth that could be perceived through the emotions: "No man can be a true Christian without such inspiration of the Holy Ghost as fills his heart with peace and joy and love, which he who perceives not has it not. This is the point for which alone I contend; and this I take to be the very foundation of Christianity."[34] This emphasis on sensible experience had much in common with the empiricism of the philosopher John Locke, though recent scholarship has suggested that John's own understanding drew on older, Aristotelian traditions.[35] Nonetheless, John Wesley agreed with Locke's contention that knowledge came from the experience of the senses rather than being innate. John's insistence on the necessity of a sensible experience of the Holy Ghost reflected a valuing of experience and observation over reasoning from first principles.[36]

Over time, however, John developed a theology of spiritual senses that distinguished him from empiricist philosophers such as Locke. John argued that God gave those who were born again a "new class of senses" with which to perceive the "invisible world" of the spirit. Such perception and the knowledge it brought were only available to those who had been born again. While this supernaturalist approach would have been unacceptable to Locke, it clearly shares much with the empiricist emphasis on the experience of the senses.

Whatever the exact relationship between John Wesley's thought and Locke's empiricist philosophy, personal experience was clearly central to early Methodist culture. The Methodist commitment to recording spiritual experience in an incredible array of literary forms, including journals, autobiographies and conversion narratives, is evidence of how significant such experience was considered.[37] These texts are not only accounts of the inner world of the emotions, they are also concerned with the external world of events, relationships and occurrences that Methodists believed were ordered by Providence. The inner world was, however, of great importance. Faith, the new birth, assurance and perfection – all must be experienced in "the heart." This emphasis on experience may help explain the attraction of Methodism to the illiterate and outcast.[38] In broader terms, it contributed to a distinctive construction of the self that had implications for Charles Wesley's understanding of the role of suffering.

The conviction that God's work could and should be felt is displayed throughout Charles Wesley's writings. In a sermon preached before the University of Oxford, he observed:

> The true, lively and converting faith, the sure and substantial faith which saveth sinners, is not only a common belief in the Articles of our creed, but it is also a true trust and confidence of the mercy of God through our Lord Jesus Christ, and a steadfast hope of all good things to be received at God's hand. It is not in the mouth and outward profession only, but liveth and stirreth in the heart.[39]

In a sermon on the Pharisee and the tax collector, Wesley drew attention to the "pattern of true repentance" displayed by the tax collector, in a description that similarly emphasized the emotional and experiential aspect of this state. The tax collector "smote upon his breast, he felt the hell of his own nature, was painfully sensible that in him dwelt no good thing, but that he was a motley mixture of beast and devil."[40]

Wesley's journals reflect his conviction that intense emotional experience was an aspect not just of conversion, but also of increasing spiritual maturity. Describing a meeting of Methodists he attended in 1744, he wrote:

> O how delightfully did we mourn after Him whom our soul loveth! Not with the noisy turbulent sorrow of newly awakened souls, which most times passes away as a morning cloud; but with the deep contrition of love; till the congregation was in tears, in silent tears of desire or joy.[41]

Given that Wesley expected the spiritual state of a person to manifest itself in emotional experience, it is not surprising to find him seeking to evoke emotion in the service of spiritual ends. Methodism was concerned with what "liveth and stirreth in the heart." Subjective responses had spiritual significance, and demanded attention and effort from the Christian.

That experience was significant with regard to hymns was suggested by John Wesley in his organization of his definitive hymnbook, *A Collection of Hymns for the Use of the People Called Methodists* (1780). John organized the hymns into sections that he claimed reflected "the experience of real Christians": sections such as "Praying for Repentance," "For Mourners Convinced of Sin," "For Believers Suffering" and "Convinced of Backsliding."[42] John's famous description of this hymnbook as "a little body of experimental and practical divinity" demonstrates the important place of hymns in establishing the relationship between experience and doctrine.[43]

It is not surprising, therefore, to find that Charles Wesley's verse is deeply concerned with the emotional world as a spiritual realm. His poems not only expressed the inner experiences of the believer but also shaped and formed them. For example, in the famous hymn originally entitled "Free Grace" (but better known as "And Can it Be?") he used questions, exclamations and a sequence of dramatic narratives to describe the conversion experience in vigorous and victorious terms (see Hymn 1). Here, it is the positive inner experiences – of personal revelation, new life and the presence of Christ in verse five, and of boldness and freedom from fear in verse six – that provide proof to the believer that the objective work of Christ has been applied to him or her. This depiction of the relationship between an outer reality and an inner response is repeated throughout Wesley's hymns and both reflected and reinforced the Methodist theology of "inward religion." But such a hymn clearly operates not only to express such experiences, but also to produce them. The questions and exclamations provoke responses of surprise and awe. The narratives draw the reader or singer into the spiritual journey of conversion: first, Christ's journey from heaven to earth and humiliation; second, the individual's journey from imprisonment and darkness to the heavenly throne. The final two lines are a spiritual act in themselves – they assume that in singing or reading these words the individual is literally approaching the throne of God.

Wesley's verse must be seen, therefore, not simply as the record of intense experience but also as a tool for interpreting and re-creating such experiences, on the assumption that they had real spiritual value. He achieved this in part through literary means, using an enormous variety of meters, metaphors and other rhetorical devices to create intense emotional effects. In studying individual hymns it is therefore crucial to pay attention to the emotional effect and intention of any work, as well as to the logic and coherency of the ideas it contains.

A focus on the emotive qualities of Wesley's verse leads to questions about a third characteristic of his work, his regular use of the first person. What is the place of the individual in Wesley's hymnody? How should the "I" and the "we" of his hymns be understood? Reading Wesley's verse as a straightforward record of his own feelings and opinions is inadequate, as even a few examples will make clear.[44] The "I" in a poem such as one entitled "Hymn for a Condemned Malefactor" is obviously vicarious.

> Suffer'd a few more hours to live,
> Before I my deserts receive,
> And justice satisfy,
> Unless my stubborn heart relent,
> Dying, unless I first repent,
> I must for ever die.[45]

By contrast, in those poems written at the time of his son Samuel's conversion to Roman Catholicism, the "I" seems much more personal and specific, a record of Wesley's own experience.

> Farewell, my all of earthly hope,
> My nature's stay, my age's prop.
> Irrevocably gone!
> Submissive to the will divine
> I acquiesce, and make it mine;
> I offer up my Son.[46]

In far more of the poems, especially those depicting the ideal spiritual states of a believer, the identity of the "I" is more general. "And Can it Be?" is typical of many hymns that describe experiences and emotions with which any devout Methodist could identify.[47]

This continual shifting of identity was both intentional and didactic.[48] In the "Hymn for a Condemned Malefactor" quoted above, Wesley was quite clearly using the first person to suggest an appropriate attitude for the malefactor to adopt, rather than trying to enter imaginatively into his or her actual attitude and thoughts. This creates the slightly odd perspective by which the "malefactor" acts as his or her own evangelist, preaching repentance to his or her own "stubborn heart."

Marshall and Todd's distinction between the "expressive *venting* of feeling" and the "evangelical *directing* of feeling" is helpful here. It is not, however, as complete a distinction as they suggest. Wesley's most personal poems, written in anguish over bereavement or betrayal, and surely a means of "venting" his feelings, display the same sense of emotions being appropriately directed. Another poem on the conversion of Wesley's son, Samuel, to Catholicism begins:

Again, my soul, to Jesus turn!
The Comforter of all that mourn,
My sorrowful request
Compassionately kind he hears,
And promises to dry my tears,
And give the weary rest.

From this self-direction of the grieving soul it moves, via a meditation on eternity, toward a statement of resignation and confident hope.

In view of such transcendent bliss,
I now my anxious grief dismiss,
My ravish'd son forego,
No more indulge my fond complaints,
No more my burthen'd Spirit faints
Beneath its hallow'd woe

I count not fit to be compar'd
To that exceeding great Reward
My light calamity,
My momentary loss and pain
Thro' which a glorious crown I gain
And God for ever see![49]

Poems such as this suggest that the process of writing allowed Wesley to express, examine and ultimately discipline his emotions into particular channels.[50] But while such an interpretation illuminates the more overtly "personal" poems, it does not explain Wesley's approach as a whole. To understand Wesley's focus on the individual, it is necessary to return to his theological convictions about the inner world as discussed above.

A notable element of all these hymns is the way in which they deliberately move the reader or singer from one emotional or spiritual state to another: from unbelief to faith; from apathy to fervor; from overwhelming grief to resignation; from faith to "speechless" ecstasy.[51] They describe a narrative of inner emotional or spiritual change.[52] For Wesley, this process of change was a matter of spiritual importance, and was necessary whether he was writing for himself or for others. Wesley's response to his own extremes of emotion seems to have been to express, shape and sanctify them through the poetic process. He was equally capable, however, of writing an exemplary display of imagined emotional change.

Attempting to establish the exact identity of the "I" in Wesley's hymns may, therefore, obscure the significance of his use of the first person.[53] The repeated use of the first person encourages the reader or singer to "own" the experience described in the hymn, interpreting it in the context of their own experience. Accompanied by the present tense, which Wesley also repeatedly used, the use of the first person places the individual at the center of a dynamic emotional process. The narrative hymns therefore reveal to us something of Wesley's inner world, but even more of how he believed that world should be interpreted and disciplined for spiritual benefit. They are essentially tools for spiritual self-formation.

Recognizing the narrative quality of Wesley's hymns links the hymns to a broader characteristic of Methodist culture. Early Methodist culture, like early evangelical culture in general, developed a central focus on the conversion narrative.[54] This "narrative culture" grew, in part, out of the Methodist valuing of experience: Methodist leaders and laypeople continually recounted their experiences of conversion as testimony to the truth of the message of justification by faith and the new birth. These narratives were communicated verbally in band meetings, written down in letters and published in John Wesley's *Arminian Magazine*. Methodism thus formed a "narrative community" within which conversion was experienced, interpreted and recounted as a story. Methodist conversion narratives tended to use particular phrases, adopt certain biblical models and follow particular patterns that distinguished them from the conversion narratives of other groups within the evangelical revivals.[55]

In his analysis of conversion narratives written in letters to Charles Wesley, D. Bruce Hindmarsh identifies hymns as playing a significant role in drawing individuals into the "narrative culture" of Methodist conversion.[56] The converts who wrote to Charles Wesley testified to the place of hymns in preparing them for the experience of conversion, in triggering the experience of the new birth and in providing a language for describing that experience. The narrative quality of the hymns makes this connection understandable. Their style and structure invited the reader or singer to rehearse the experience of conversion, and provided a narrative within which the reader or singer could place their own experience.

Hymns, however, contained narratives not only of conversion, but also of spiritual experiences in every state of life, including suffering. They point to the existence of a broader Methodist narrative culture, in which every event of life mattered and could be interpreted within a story of spiritual significance.[57] In particular, the inner life of the emotions had to be observed and tended. The hymns provided Methodists with a tool for expressing and directing their experiences and their emotions for spiritual benefit. As individuals read or sang Wesley's hymns, therefore, they were encouraged to focus on the "inner world" of the heart, understanding it as the moral and spiritual center of the self.

Wesley's Use of Hymns

The ways in which Wesley used the hymns in his daily life and ministry confirm that he understood the hymns in these terms. His letters and journal reveal that hymn-singing and reading were an intrinsic feature of his daily life, as well as his ministry. As he itinerated around the country, Wesley and his companions sang hymns constantly, alone and together. Aboard ship for a day on one journey: "We spent the day in singing and reading."[58] In Wales, on another occasion, he was met by a group of Methodist women and recorded: "We went on our way singing and rejoicing."[59] Traveling in Ireland, he described overtaking "a lad whistling one of our tunes. He was a constant hearer, though a Roman, and joined with us in several hymns which he had by heart."[60]

Hymn-singing was, for Wesley, the appropriate response to any event of spiritual significance. After surviving fierce anti-Methodist riots in Bristol, he recorded that he and the other Methodist itinerants "joined in hearty praises to our Deliverer, singing the hymn, – 'Worship, and thanks, and blessing.'"[61] On hearing of the death of a Methodist: "We sang a song of victory for our deceased friend, then went to the house and rejoiced, and gave thanks: and rejoiced again with singing over him."[62] Following his success in refuting charges of treason at Wakefield in 1744, the "brethren met us on the road, and we gathered together on the hill, and sang praises lustily, with a good courage."[63]

As contemporary critics noted, hymns were distinctive of Methodist meetings of all kinds.[64] Hymn-singing was often prolonged. On one occasion, Wesley recorded his disappointment that opposition from the crowd during an open-air meeting meant "we could only sing for half an hour."[65] At a watchnight service: "We sang together, and shouted for joy, till morning."[66] Wesley's accounts show that hymns provided a means for the congregation to express – perhaps spontaneously – their reactions to the service. "In the midst of my discourse," he recorded of one meeting, "we all broke out into joy and singing."[67] A more spectacular incident demonstrates how hymn-singing could provide flexible and emotionally powerful tools for the preacher:

> From those words, "I will that they may behold my glory," while I was speaking of our Lord's appearing, we were alarmed with the loudest clap of thunder I ever heard... Most of the congregation shrieked out, as if the day of the Lord were come. A thought darted into my heart as quick as lightning, "What if it should be the day of judgment!" I was filled immediately with faith, stronger than death, and rejoiced in hope of the glory of God. The same spirit rested on all the faithful, while I broke out into singing
> So shall the Lord the Saviour come,
> And lightnings round his chariot play!
> Ye lightnings, fly to make him room,
> Ye glorious storms prepare his way![68]

Wesley's immediate choice of a hymn (rather than, for example, a prayer or an exhortation) to respond to this unexpected event demonstrates the significance of hymns in the drama of the Methodist meeting.

The potential value of hymns in responding to unexpected developments during Methodist meetings is also demonstrated in Wesley's account of a meeting in Bristol. The Calvinist Howel Harris (a close friend of Wesley's notwithstanding their theological differences) had been invited to preach. Harris's sermon extolled the Calvinist doctrine of irresistible grace and, after some time, Wesley interrupted the sermon to ask the listening Society whether they wished to hear any more. The Society indicated that they did not.

> Howel Harris would have entered into dispute, but was stopped. "Then," said he, "you thrust me out." "No," said I, "we do not: you are welcome to stay as long as you please. We acknowledge you a child of God." Yet again he began, "If you do not believe irresistible grace;" and I cut off the sentence of reprobation which I foresaw coming, with,
> Praise God from whom pure blessings flow,
> Whose bowels yearn on *all* below;
> Who would not have one sinner lost;
> Praise Father, Son and Holy Ghost.[69]

Here again Wesley used a hymn (in this case a re-writing of the doxology with an Arminian emphasis) to respond to an unexpected situation within the meeting and, presumably, to encourage the faithful to join with him in the appropriate response.

Wesley also used hymns in his pastoral work, and it is his accounts of these situations that demonstrate how powerful hymns could be in more personal contexts. In a letter to a Methodist widow, he included a hymn entitled "The Widow's Hymn" and urged her to pass it on to any to whom it was relevant. "Great fellowship I have," he added, "with widows that are widows indeed."[70] The hymn that Wesley included begins, "O Thou, who plead'st the Widow's Cause/ Who only canst repair my loss" and is clearly designed for the devotional use of widows. Similarly, Wesley wrote to his wife, Sally, during one of her pregnancies, enquiring: "Are you much in private prayer? Do you ever read my hymns for your condition?"[71] Here he was presumably referring to his hymns for women "in Travail."[72] As his letter makes clear, while Wesley described these poems as hymns, he expected them to be read rather than sung.

In a more striking example of his use of the hymns with individuals, in his journal Wesley recorded counseling a woman who had experienced conversion but was afraid to admit it. He asked her to join in singing the first verse of one of his hymns, "O Filial Deity," which concluded, "Take me now, possess me whole,/ Who for me, for me hast died." While singing the last line, Wesley wrote, "she burst out into tears and outcries, 'I believe, I believe!' and sunk down. She continued and increased in the assurance of faith; full of peace, and joy, and hope."[73]

These accounts of Wesley's experiences suggest that he used hymns in a wide variety of contexts, as a flexible spiritual tool. His hymn-writing was presumably informed by this experience. By providing narratives of spiritual change that directed individual emotion in particular directions, Wesley's hymns could act as tools for personal devotion, congregational song, exhortation, testimony or pastoral counseling. His experience of finding that hymns were effective – and popular – for these ends, surely reinforced his understanding of hymns in these terms.[74]

This interpretation of Wesley's hymns illuminates elements that also appeared in the sentimental novels of the eighteenth century. Just as the heroes and heroines of eighteenth-century novels demonstrated to readers the correct responses to moral dilemmas, so Wesley's hymns modeled ideal spiritual attitudes and reactions.[75] While there are significant similarities between the narratives of spiritual change in Wesley's hymns and the narratives of moral improvement in the novels of Richardson and other eighteenth-century novelists, the differences between these genres are also instructive. The reading or singing of a hymn could directly involve the reader or singer to a degree that a novel – or such traditional forms of moral instruction as the sermon – could not. A hymn, with its rhythm, rhyme and (relative) brevity, was designed to be remembered and repeated, continually re-affirming a particular idea or emotional process. The participation of the reader or singer was further encouraged by the use of the first person in the text, even more so where the hymn was written for a specific group (such as widows). The similarities between Wesley's hymns and "sentimental literature" do point, however, to the importance of the broader cultural context of eighteenth-century England within which these genres developed. Both genres reflect a Lockean interest in sensible experience.

This comparison also draws attention to the question of gender in the hymns. In her study of early American Methodism, Diane Lobody concludes that the movement "spoke a woman's language": "Over and again, with almost ritual intonation, we hear the language of tender and uncontrollable emotionalism – the language of women's nature and behaviour."[76] The hymns, with their depiction of emotional responsiveness to God, put this language into the mouths of all believers, regardless of sex. This emphasis on emotional sensitivity was accompanied by more conventionally masculine language, referring to power and conflict.[77] In singing or reading the hymns, women applied this imagery to themselves, and so gender boundaries were blurred in more ways than one. Wesley's emphasis on emotional responsiveness, however, reflected a broader trend in eighteenth-century literature to construct the ideal man or woman as highly emotionally sensitive, in terms that would increasingly be criticized as effeminate.[78] While gender is not a central category of my analysis, the connections between Wesley's hymns and this "literature of sensibility," as well as the wider implications of his use of language for questions of gender in early Methodism, will be considered at several points in the following chapters.

Reading Wesley's Hymns

In reading Wesley's verse, then, it is important to be sensitive to differences in genre and context of writing, and to the ways in which these differences may affect the content of the verse. It is also important to be aware that his verse does not simply make objective statements to the reader or singer, but draws the reader in as a participant in an emotional process that is given profound spiritual significance. When reading one of Wesley's hymns, it is necessary to ask, not just "What does it say?" but also "What does it do?"

This approach provides a framework both for considering Wesley's treatment of suffering in his poetical writings and for re-evaluating Wesley's significance to the Methodist movement more broadly. It places suffering in a wider context of emotional experiences that Charles was concerned to explore. John's response to his brother's poetry shows that Charles's insistent focus on pain and emotional struggle went beyond what John considered appropriate. Nonetheless, the conviction that emotions were significant explains Charles's determination to see spiritual meaning in even his most agonized feelings and his decision to express those feelings in poetry presented for public use.

More importantly, the recognition that so many of Wesley's hymns were designed as a means of personal change leads to a particular understanding of the ways in which they engage with the experience of suffering. Wesley's hymns do reveal his theology of suffering but, more immediately, they also demonstrate his construction of the experience of suffering: of what he understood suffering to consist, how he thought it should be managed, what its spiritual and personal uses were. This awareness encourages particular attention to be paid to the cultural resources upon which Wesley drew in making sense of, and managing, the experience of suffering.

Wesley's hymns provided a means by which Methodists could construct their own experience of suffering for spiritual benefit. Methodism developed a powerful "narrative culture" and Wesley's hymns contributed to this culture. Understanding the role of Charles Wesley's hymns in these terms provides a new perspective on Wesley's significance within early Methodism. Historians and theologians have considered his undeniable contribution to the movement in terms of his efforts as preacher, pastor and ecclesiastical politician. They have noted the ways in which his hymns promoted particular doctrines and formed the liturgical culture of the Methodist movement. This chapter suggests that Charles Wesley's influence on early Methodism must be sought beyond his contributions as activist, theologian and liturgist, within the shape of early Methodist experience.

It is beyond the scope of this study to establish the exact nature of the relationship between the hymns and early Methodist culture: this would require further analysis of Methodist practice and reception studies of the kind that have only recently been attempted with regard to Wesley's hymns.[79] Instead, by analyzing the letters and journals of early Methodists in conjunction with the hymns, the following chapters suggest ways in which early Methodist perceptions of suffering reflected – or resisted – the construction of suffering encouraged by the hymns they read and sang.[80] In so doing, it contributes to broader debates about the nature of early Methodist culture.

Reading his brother's hymns *in memoriam*, John Wesley was struck by the "gloomy cast" of Charles's verses and his mind. For John, this was evidence of a spiritual problem, the residue of the "poisonous mysticism" that had once so attracted both brothers. The hymns were not, however, simply the personal reflections of one individual, but a tool for constructing the Christian self. Charles's "melancholy" view of religion was significant not only for his own experience, but also for the experience of the thousands who read and sang his hymns. His hymns about suffering were works that both constructed and managed the painful experiences they represented.

[Hymn 1]
Free Grace

1. And can it be, that I should gain
An interest in the Saviour's blood?
Died he for me, who caused His pain?
For me? Who Him to death pursued?
Amazing love! How can it be
That Thou, my God, shouldst die for me?

2. 'Tis myst'ry all: th'Immortal dies!
Who can explore His strange design?
In vain the first-born seraph tries
To sound the depths of love divine.
'Tis mercy all! Let earth adore!
Let angel minds inquire no more.

3. He left His Father's throne above
(So free, so infinite His grace!)
Emptied Himself of all but love,
And bled for Adam's helpless race,
'Tis mercy all, immense and free,
For, O my God, it found out me!

4. Long my imprisoned spirit lay,
Fast bound in sin and nature's night.
Thine eye diffused a quick'ning ray;
I woke; the dungeon flamed with light.
My chains fell off, my heart was free,
I rose, went forth, and followed Thee.

5. Still the small inward voice I hear,
That whispers all my sins forgiven;
Still the atoning blood is near,
That quench'd the wrath of hostile Heaven:
I feel the life His wounds impart;
I feel my Saviour in my heart.

6. No condemnation now I dread,
Jesus, and all in Him, is mine.
Alive in Him, my living head,
And clothed in righteousness divine,
Bold I approach th'eternal throne,
And claim the crown, through Christ my own.[81]

Notes

1. 15 Dec. 1788. W. R. Ward and Richard P. Heitzenrater, eds., *Journal and Diaries VII (1787–91)*, vol. 24, *BEW* (Nashville: Abingdon Press, 2003), 117. Here, mean" implies "average" rather than "poor."

2. 28 June 1788. *BEW*, 24: 97.

3. "Introduction," in *Framing and Imagining Disease in Cultural History*, ed. George Sebastian Rousseau, Miranda Gill, David Haycock and Malte Herwig (Basingstoke, Hampshire: Palgrave Macmillan, 2003), 14.

4. This outline makes use of the lists of Charles Wesley's works in *UP* 1: 11–15; Frank Baker, *Representative Verse of Charles Wesley* (London: Epworth Press, 1962), 379–94; Telford, *The Life of the Rev. Charles Wesley, M.A.*, 311–13.

5. See Henry Bett, *The Hymns of Methodism* (London: Epworth Press, 1945), 25–26; Tyson, ed., *Charles Wesley*, 29.

6. Baker, *Charles Wesley's Verse*, 105.

7. John Wesley to Elizabeth Ritchie, 1786, quoted by Rack, *Reasonable Enthusiast*, 548–49.

8. Albert C. Outler cautions against accepting John Wesley's (repeated) description of himself as rarely in low spirits. Both early and late in his life he wrote letters describing emotions close to despair. These were, however, far rarer than Charles's depressions. See Albert C. Outler, ed., *Sermons II*, vol. 2, *BEW* (Nashville: Abingdon Press, 1984), 202–4.

9. John did write an intensely emotional verse account of his relationship with Grace Murray in 1749. *BEW*, 2: 264.

10. John Wesley, "The Wilderness State," *BEW* 2: 219.

11. Frank Baker argues, "Charles's writing tended to be exuberant and unrestrained, while John's was severe and sober." Baker, *Charles Wesley's Verse*, 105.

12. John made the "namby-pambical" comment in a letter to Charles, 26 Dec. 1761. John Wesley, *The Works of John Wesley*, 14 vols., vol. 12 (Grand Rapids: Zondervan, 1958), 122. He criticized the use of "fondling expression" in his sermon "On Knowing Christ After the Flesh," Albert C. Outler, ed., *Sermons IV*, vol. 4, *BEW* (Nashville: Abingdon Press, 1987), 102–3.

13. For examples of John's editing decisions, see Baker, *Representative Verse*, 37, 58, 67, 88, 100, 25.

14. John Wesley, "On Knowing Christ after the Flesh," *BEW* 4: 102–3.

15. John Wesley, "On Knowing Christ after the Flesh," *BEW* 4: 102.

16. As discussed in Chapter Four, John Wesley did preach a number of sermons exploring the experience of "heaviness" or depression.

17. John Wesley, "A Plain Account of Christian Perfection." Wesley, *The Works of John Wesley*, 11: 391.

18. *SHSPHS* (1762): "Preface." *PW* 9: vii.

19. John Wesley to Dorothy Furly, 15 Sept. 1762. Wesley, *The Works of John Wesley*, 12: 207. In the context, John is clearly referring to Charles's portrayal of the doctrine of perfection. The difference between the brothers on this question, and its significance for their understanding of suffering, is discussed in Chapter Four.

20. Some of these poems were published in edited or altered forms during his lifetime. Others, such as "funeral hymns," were written for public use and would probably have been sung and disseminated even if not published. For further discussion of Charles Wesley's funeral hymns, see Chapter Six.

21. F. Luke Wiseman, *Charles Wesley: Evangelist and Poet* (London: Epworth Press, 1932), 199.

22. Marshall and Todd, *English Congregational Hymns*, 1, 7.

23. Marshall and Todd, *English Congregational Hymns*, 79. Emphasis mine.

24. *UP* 1: 231–32.

25. *SHSPHS* (1762): "1 Sam. 1: 23." *PW* 9: 149.

26. Richard Arnold, *The English Hymn: Studies in a Genre* (New York: Peter Lang, 1995), 1.

27. For example, Bishop Ken's Morning and Evening hymns, the hymns of George Withers, or John Donne's "Hymne to God the Father," which Donne had sung by the choristers of St. Paul's at Evening Service. See J. R. Watson, *The English Hymn: A Critical and Historical Study* (Oxford: Clarendon Press, 1997), 57–80; Susan S. Tarnke, *Make a Joyful Noise Unto the Lord* (Ohio: Ohio University Press, 1978), 17.

28. Arnold, *The English Hymn*, 65–78.

29. *The Monthly Review*, 1762. Quoted in Arnold, *The English Hymn*, 78.

30. Between 1741 and 1780, the number of English language hymnbooks being published per decade doubled. Mark A. Noll, "The Defining Role of Hymns in Early Evangelicalism," in *Wonderful Words of Life: Hymns in American Protestant History and Theology*, ed. Richard J. Mouw and Mark A. Noll (Grand Rapids: William B. Eerdmans, 2004), 7.

31. Davie, *The Eighteenth-Century Hymn in England*, 57.

32. *Hymns for the Nativity of our Lord* (1745): "Hymn IV." *PW* 4: 108.

33. For example, Frederick Dreyer, "Faith and Experience in the Thought of John Wesley," *The American Historical Review* 88, no. 1 (1983): 12–30; Richard E. Brantley, *Locke, Wesley and the Method of English Romanticism* (Gainesville: University Presses of Florida, 1984); David Hempton, *Methodism: Empire of the Spirit* (New Haven and London: Yale University Press, 2005), 32–54; Rack, *Reasonable Enthusiast*, 384–88; Gregory S. Clapper, *John Wesley on Religious Affections: His Views on Experience and Emotion and Their Role in the Christian Life and Theology* (Metuchen, N.J., and London: Scarecrow Press, Inc., 1989).

34. John Wesley, *The Letters of the Rev. John Wesley, A.M., Sometime Fellow of Lincoln College, Oxford* ed. John Telford, 8 vols. (London: 1931), 2: 64. Quoted in Dreyer, "Faith and Experience," 15.

35. Dreyer, "Faith and Experience," 15. For a discussion of recent challenges to the claim that John Wesley took his empiricist views from Locke, see Rebecca Irelan, "A Little Experiment in Practical Divinity: Charles Sanders Peirce and the Women of Early Methodism Socialize the Subject of John Wesley's Doctrine of Sanctification" (PhD diss., Graduate Theological Union, 2008), 80–83.

36. This did not mean that feelings were the final arbiter of truth: the Wesleys recognized the overarching authority of Scripture and the lesser authorities of church tradition and reason. Jean-Pierre van Noppen, *Transforming Words: The Early Methodist Revival from a Discourse Perspective* (Bern: Peter Lang, 1999), 122–23.

37. Hempton, *Methodism*, 52.

38. John Walsh, "'Methodism' and the Origins of English-Speaking Evangelicalism," in *Evangelicalism: Comparative Studies of Popular Protestantism in North America, the British Isles, and Beyond, 1700–1990*, ed. Mark A. Noll, David W. Bebbington, and George A. Rawlyk (New York, Oxford: Oxford University Press, 1994), 31.

39. Sermon 7: Romans 3: 23–25. Newport, ed., *Sermons*, 200–201.

40. Sermon 12: Luke 18: 9–14. Newport, ed. *Sermons*, 272.

41. 11 Aug. 1744. *CWJ* 1: 400.

42. Franz Hildebrandt and Oliver A Beckerlegge, eds., *A Collection of Hymns for the Use of the People Called Methodists*, vol. 7, *BEW* (Oxford: Clarendon Press, 1983), 77–78.

43. *BEW*, 7: 74.

44. For example, Richard E. Brantley, "Charles Wesley's Experiential Art," *Eighteenth-Century Life* 11, no. 2 (1987): 1–11.

45. "Hymn for a Condemned Malefactor." *UP* 3: 317.

46. *UP* 1: 304.

47. *HSP* (1740): "Groaning for the Spirit of Adoption." *PW* 1: 307.

48. Baker, *Representative Verse*, xvi–xvii.

49. ["Hymns on his son Samuel, Hymn VI"] *UP* 1: 306–7.

50. Shields, "Charles Wesley as Poet," 65.

51. This quality of emotional "movement" in Methodist hymns is also noted by van Noppen, *Transforming Words*, 212.

52. Susan Wise Bauer distinguishes helpfully between "narrative" and "systematic" hymns in "Stories and Syllogisms: Protestant Hymns, Narrative Theology, and Heresy," in *Wonderful Words of Life*, eds. Mouw and Noll, 208, 216.

53. Watson, *The English Hymn: A Critical and Historical Study*, 20.

54. Hindmarsh, 153.

55. Hindmarsh, *The Evangelical Conversion Narrative*, 63–64, 128, 324.

56. Hindmarsh, *The Evangelical Conversion Narrative*, 153.

57. In his analysis, Hindmarsh focuses on the experience of conversion, but he notes that in the letters to Charles Wesley "conversion appears as a special case of the more general category of spiritual experience that Wesley wished to record and preserve." Hindmarsh, *The Evangelical Conversion Narrative*, 131.

58. 13 Aug. 1745. *CWJ* 1: 403.

59. 11 Aug. 1744. *CWJ* 1: 377.

60. 8 Feb. 1748. *CWJ* 2: 2.

61. 25 Feb. 1747. *CWJ* 1: 449.

62. 14 Aug. 1744. *CWJ* 1: 378–79.

63. 15 Mar. 1744. *CWJ* 1: 362.

64. Van Noppen, *Transforming Words*, 67.

65. 30 Nov. 1744. *CWJ* 1: 389.

66. 31 May 1745. *CWJ* 1: 398.

67. 18 Jan. 1747. *CWJ* 1: 440.

68. 23 June 1745. *CWJ* 1: 400.

69. 28 June 1741. *CWJ* 1: 284. Emphasis in original.

70. Charles Wesley to Elizabeth Witham, 16 Jan. [1746]. DDCW 1/14a.

71. Charles Wesley to Sally Wesley, 29 Apr. [nd]. DDCW 5/87.

72. Twenty hymns for women "in Travail" were published in *Hymns for the Use of Families* (1767). *PW* 7: 54–65. For further discussion of these hymns, see Chapter Five.

73. 2 July 1738. *CWJ* 1: 115.

74. While this analysis has focused on Wesley's use of the hymns, letters written by Methodists often refer to hymns being used in a wide variety of contexts. See, for example, Thomas Middleton to Charles Wesley, 8 Oct. 1743. EMV 111; Mary Jane Ramsey to Charles Wesley, 4 June 1740. EMV 13; Fanny Cowper to Charles Wesley, 8 March 1741. EMV 43; Elizabeth Sais to Charles Wesley, May 1742. EMV 126. See also "Account of Executions," [nd]. EMV 141.

75. Marshall and Todd, *English Congregational Hymns*, 11.

76. D. H. Lobody, "'That language might be given me': Women's experience in early Methodism," in *Perspectives on American Methodism: Interpretive Essays*, ed. E. Richey (Nashville: Abingdon Press, 1993), 141.

77. For a discussion of gender and language in the hymns, see van Noppen, *Transforming Words*, 116–17.

78. For extensive analysis of this cultural trend, see G. J. Barker-Benfield, *The Culture of Sensibility: Sex and Society in Eighteenth-Century Britain* (Chicago: University of Chicago Press, 1992).

79. For example, Stephen Marini has compiled statistics on the frequency with which particular hymns were published among evangelicals, as a way of judging what evangelicals actually sang. See Stephen Marini, "Hymnody as History: Early Evangelical Hymns and the Recovery of American Popular Religion," *Church History* 71, no. 2 (2002): 273–307. For a broader discussion of "discourse reception" with regard to early Methodism, see van Noppen, *Transforming Words*, 162–68.

80. In particular, I use the collections of letters written to Charles Wesley, found in the EMV and DDWES collections within the Methodist Archives and Research Centre, as well as the personal writings of early Methodist women within the Fletcher-Tooth Collection (F/T) in the same location. I also refer to Paul Wesley Chilcote, ed., *Her Own Story: Autobiographical Portraits of Early Methodist Women* (Nashville, Tenn.: Kingswood Books, 2001) and John Wesley, *Letters*, ed. Frank Baker, vol. 25–26, *BEW* (Nashville: Abingdon, 1976–).

81. *HSP* (1739). *PW* 1: 105–6.

Chapter Three

Sorrow, Sight and Transformation

On 10 July 1738, Charles Wesley recorded in his journal that he had begun visiting ten condemned men imprisoned in Newgate. It was less than two months after his conversion experience and he visited the men with reluctance: "My old prejudices against the possibility of a death-bed repentance still hung upon me; and I could hardly hope there was mercy for those whose time was so short."[1] In the prison he met a "poor black" sentenced to death for stealing from his master:

> I told him of One who came down from heaven to save lost sinners, and him in particular; described the sufferings of the Son of God, his sorrows, agony, and death. He listened with all the signs of eager astonishment; the tears trickled down his cheeks, while he cried, "What! was it for me? Did God suffer all this for so poor a creature as me?" I left him waiting for the salvation of God.[2]

Other prisoners responded to Wesley's preaching with similar emotion. Later that week, while spending the night locked in Newgate with them, Wesley led them in singing a hymn his father had written with the title "On the Crucifixion." The hymn began with the words:

> Behold the Saviour of mankind,
> Nail'd to the sinful tree!
> How vast the love that him inclined,
> To bleed and die for thee.[3]

On 19 July, following the conversion of all ten men, Wesley accompanied them to their execution at Tyburn. Waiting at the gallows, the men again joined in singing "On the Crucifixion." Wesley noted: "They were all cheerful; full of comfort, peace, and triumph; assuredly persuaded Christ had died for them, and waited to receive them into paradise."[4]

In Wesley's account, the description of the "sufferings of the Son of God" is transformative for the men who listen to it. In the first instance, the sufferings of Jesus produce "eager astonishment," tears and repentance in the "poor black" who hears them described. In the second, the sufferings of Jesus, described again in the words of Samuel Wesley's hymn, are used to encourage the ten men to accept cheerfully their own suffering and deaths. This account makes an appropriate introduction to an analysis of the meaning and power of Christ's suffering in Wesley's hymns. Wesley's construction of the Passion forms the interpretive key to much of his broader portrayal of suffering.

The Atonement

In Christian theology "the atonement" has generally been used to refer to the work or achievement of Christ in his life, death and resurrection, with "theories of the atonement" denoting alternative interpretations of this work.[5] Others have discussed Wesley's doctrine of the atonement at length and in detail: this analysis is concerned with the way in which he understood suffering within this theological framework.[6] Historically, many theories of the atonement have been proffered by theologians, incorporating a range of biblical themes and images. These theories can be grouped with relation to four central themes: sacrifice, victory, forgiveness and moral example.[7] Wesley's broader doctrine of the atonement makes use of all of these themes, a diversity that is not surprising given the broad context of his theological development: an upbringing in a strictly High Church of England family, a formal theological education at Oxford, intense devotional reading of mystic writers and close contact with German pietists. Within this diversity, however, two concepts (related in Wesley's thought) are particularly relevant to his interpretation of Christ's suffering: penal substitution and recapitulation. These two ideas relate particularly to the theological themes of sacrifice and forgiveness, and form the essential context of his expression of the meaning and power of Christ's suffering.

Wesley's theological statements demonstrate his acceptance of the concept of penal substitution, or substitutionary atonement. This doctrine, traceable in its initial formulation to Anselm of Canterbury (c. 1033–1109) and reformulated by the Reformers in the sixteenth century, relies on the idea that God's justice is deeply offended by human sinfulness. Christ's death is the event in which God's justice was satisfied: Christ, who was both God and perfect man, died in the place of humanity, and accomplished the propitiation of God's wrath against sin. Human beings are now able to participate in the ensuing benefits.[8] This interpretation of Christ's death lends itself particularly to the use of imagery of Old Testament rituals of sacrifice, in which unblemished animals were offered to atone for human sin. On several occasions Wesley quoted approvingly from the Church of England homily "On Salvation" to support his view:

> [I]t is our duty ever to remember the great mercy of God, how that (all the world being wrapped in sin by breaking of the law) God sent his only Son our Saviour Jesus Christ into the world, to fulfill the law for us, and by the shedding of his most precious blood, to make a sacrifice and satisfaction or amends to his Father for our sins, and assuage his wrath and indignation conceived against us for the same.[9]

The idea of penal substitution also appears repeatedly throughout Wesley's hymns. An example is a hymn on Mark 15: 25.

> 1. Prostrate, with eyes of faith I see
> My Saviour fasten'd to the tree,
> A victim on that altar laid,
> Himself presenting to the skies,
> The grand vicarious sacrifice.
> The Righteous in the sinner's stead.
>
> 2. Well-pleasing to our God above,
> His sacrifice of life and love
> I plead before the gracious throne:
> Father, a prodigal receive,
> And bid a pardon'd rebel live,
> The purchase of Thy bleeding Son.[10]

The language of substitutionary atonement used here – of sacrifice, substitution, human rebellion and grace – can be seen again and again in Wesley's hymns.

For Wesley, as for other evangelicals, substitutionary atonement was the basis for the important doctrine of justification by faith. Christ's death provided the means by which human beings could receive forgiveness from God and be justified. The individual received this benefit through faith. As Wesley contended in a sermon, the moment in which a sinner looked to Christ in faith was the same moment in which that sinner was healed: "his sins are forgiven, his person is accepted, his faith hath made him whole."[11]

The atonement became effective for the individual through faith, as the individual was justified before God and received the inner change that was the new birth.[12] Wesley described this process as "receiving the atonement." A Methodist believer described her experience of receiving the atonement in answer to Wesley's questions:

> I... asked, "Has God then bestowed faith upon you?" "Yes, he has." "Why, have you peace with God?" "Yes, perfect peace." "And do you love Christ above all things?" "I do, above all things incomparably." "Then you are willing to die?" "I am, and would be glad to die this moment; for I know all my sins are blotted out; the handwriting that was against me is taken out of the way, and nailed to his cross. He has saved me by his death; he has washed me with his blood; he has hid me in his wounds. I have peace in Him, and rejoice with joy unspeakable, and full of glory." Her answers were so full to these and the most searching questions I could ask, that I had no doubt of her having received the atonement.[13]

As was noted in the previous chapter, Methodists believed that personal experience had spiritual significance. While the atonement was conceived as an objective reality, achieved by Jesus at a particular point in history, it was the subjective experience of the individual that indicated that the benefits of the atonement had been personally appropriated or received.[14]

In both Wesley's hymns and other Methodist writings, "blood" became a common shorthand term signifying Christ's sacrificial work. "Blood" is the most common soteriological term in Wesley's hymns. It appears nearly 800 times in the later hymns, which is around twice the number of occurrences in the Authorized Version used in Wesley's time.[15] A hymn responding to Jeremiah 8: 22 ("Is there no balm in Gilead?") uses the term repeatedly:

Yes, there is, there is, my God,
Balm, abundant balm in Thee,
Rivers of atoning blood,
Streams of living purity!
Pour the blood upon my soul,
Plunge me in the cleansing wave,
Close my wounds, and make me whole,
Show forth all Thy skill to save.[16]

In just eight lines, blood heals, atones, cleanses and baptizes. As in this poem, much of Wesley's use of the word "blood" elsewhere is metaphorical. By employing this word so frequently, however, he repeatedly drew attention to the physical realities of Christ's death in a way that, as will be seen, reflected his understanding of the importance of the physical suffering of Christ.

A second aspect of Wesley's doctrine of the atonement is the concept of recapitulation.[17] This concept relies on a series of parallels, in which Adam represents all of sinful humanity, whereas Christ represents those who are redeemed. The fall of Adam is seen as resulting in the loss of the image of God (moral perfection) in all mankind. The goal of God's work in human history is therefore to restore this image in humanity. Christ achieved this by being perfect himself, and making it possible by his sacrifice for humans to be forgiven and begin the journey toward perfection. An early sermon, written by John Wesley but copied and repeatedly preached by Charles, emphasized that the "one thing now needful" for individuals was to "recover our first estate, from which we are thus fallen, is the one thing now needful – to re-exchange the image of Satan for the image of God, bondage for freedom, sickness for health."[18] While this sermon dates from the early days of Wesley's ministry, the idea of Christ as the second Adam, bringing about the possible re-formation of the image of God in humanity, was to remain a constant theme in his hymns.[19]

For Wesley, the concept of recapitulation provided an overarching context within which Christ's substitutionary death could be understood. Wesley related these ideas to one another in a lengthy hymn entitled "Jesus Christ, the Saviour of all men." After describing Christ's prayer of forgiveness on the cross, the hymn continues:

13. He prays for those that shed His blood:
And who from Jesu's blood is pure?
Who hath not crucified his God?
Whose sins did not His death procure?
If all have sinn'd through *Adam's* fall,
Our Second *Adam* died for all.

14. *Adam* descended from above
Our loss of *Eden* to retrieve,
Great God of universal love,
If all the world in Thee *may* live,
In us a quickening Spirit be,
And witness, Thou hast died for me.

15. Extend to me the cleansing tide
Which freely flow'd for all mankind,
Open the fountain of Thy side,
In Thee may I redemption find,
Give *me* redemption in Thy blood;
For me and all mankind it flow'd.[20]

Here Christ is portrayed as both the substitute for the individual sinner and the representative of all humanity. The benefits of his death include both personal forgiveness and the restoration of a perfect world, or Eden.

Wesley's soteriology does, of course, contain many theological concepts other than those mentioned here – for example, the idea of Christ's death as a ransom paid to God and an Arminian emphasis on the universal scope of the atonement are two that figure throughout his poetic descriptions of Christ's death. It is in Wesley's exploration of substitutionary atonement and recapitulation, however, that much of his focus on Christ's suffering is found. In this context, Wesley made it clear that he understood Christ's sufferings to be central to the meaning of his death, and thus to its benefits for humanity.

The Atonement and Suffering

Wesley's sermons and hymns contain straightforward statements about the nature of the atonement. Both also make reference to the significance of Christ's suffering within this doctrine. In the sermons, however, the references to Christ's sufferings are only brief. In one of his sermons, Wesley described the repentance of a poor publican in these terms:

> I deserve a thousand hells; but Christ has taken my deserts and given me his. He was made sin for me, who knew no sin, that I might be made the righteousness of God in him. He came to seek and save that which was lost. He is the physician of them that be sick, the friend, the saviour and advocate of sinners. *He suffered for the unjust: I am unjust.* He died for sinners: I am a sinner! He justifies the ungodly: I am ungodly![21]

Here Christ's suffering is a parallel term for his death and its justifying effects. It is the same in a sermon on the woman caught in adultery: "Believe this, Oh thou chief of sinners; *believe he suffered once for all,* the just for the unjust; he tasted death for every man; he loved thee and gave himself for thee."[22]

In these passages, which are typical of Wesley's few references to Christ's suffering in his sermons, he did not elaborate on the details or the meaning of this suffering. In both instances, however, Christ's suffering is used as a parallel term for his death, and its justifying effects, pointing to the close relationship Wesley saw between them. Perhaps significantly, both references occur in contexts where he was clearly seeking to evoke in his listeners an affective response to what Christ has done. In addition, the account given by Wesley of his message to the "poor black" suggests that his extempore preaching often included descriptions of the sufferings of Christ.

Unlike the extant sermons, Wesley's hymns are full of references to Christ's sufferings, revealing in far more detail his understanding of the significance of these sufferings. A poetic commentary on the curse on Adam found in Genesis 3: 17–19 places Christ's sufferings within this broader framework.

1. Most righteous God, my doom I bear,
My load of guilt, and pain, and care,
Enslaved to base desires,
Hard-toiling for embitter'd bread,
I mourn my barren soul o'erspread
With cursed thorns and briars.

2. Death's sentence in myself receive,
And dust, to dust already cleave,
Exiled from paradise,
Hastening to hellish misery,
Jesus, if unredeem'd by Thee,
My soul forever dies.

3. But Jesus hath our sentence borne,
He did in our affliction mourn,
A man of sorrows made,
A servant and a curse for me;
He bears the utmost penalty,
He suffers in my stead.

4. I see Him sweat great drops of blood,
I see Him faint beneath my load!
The thorns His temples tear!
He bows His bleeding head and dies!
He lives! He mounts above the skies,
He claims my *Eden* there![23]

The poem emphasizes the spiritual state of the sinner by making the experience of this curse partly metaphorical – it is the soul of the sinner that is "o'erspread/ With cursed thorns and briars." Verses three and four then mirror the first two by portraying Christ bearing Adam's curse to redeem humanity. Significantly, he does so not only in his death but also through his suffering – and since his death is barely mentioned, mainly through his suffering. The details that Wesley chose to mention – Christ's sweating of blood at Gethsemane, his collapsing under the load of the cross, his wearing of the crown of thorns – are clearly intended to parallel the details of the curse. They indicate that Jesus is bearing the curse of human suffering – life outside paradise – as well as death. Through bearing this curse as the second Adam, Jesus is able to restore Eden.

The same understanding of Christ's suffering, in which he suffers as the second Adam, can be seen in a number of Wesley's hymns. Different aspects of Christ's experience are taken to represent different aspects of the sin and judgment of Adam. For example, in the following hymn Wesley commented on the flogging of Jesus, as described in John 19.

> The Man of griefs by all despised,
> Loaded with pain and infamy,
> Like a rebellious slave chastised,
> We mourn but wonder not to see:
> He stands in the first *Adam's* place
> Beneath our penalties and pains,
> Of all our disobedient race
> The sin and chastisement sustains.[24]

Christ's flogging – a standard punishment for a slave – is an appropriate punishment for one who represents rebellious humanity. Another hymn provides a similar interpretation of Christ sweating blood before his death. Just as Adam was sentenced to "a common sweat below," so "Jesus, to retrieve our loss,/ Sorer toil must undergo:/ While he all our sins sustains."[25] Again, this hymn suggests that Christ's suffering is included in his representative atonement for humanity. Suffering, not simply death, is necessary for his redemptive work.

Wesley interpreted Christ's suffering within the framework of recapitulation, but he also emphasized, in line with his understanding of penal substitution, that this suffering was the direct result of God's judgment on human sinfulness. Each individual sinner could therefore be held responsible for Christ's suffering. Wesley wrote in one hymn:

> 1. To Him we have nail'd to the tree
> We look, and in bitterness mourn!
> The wounds were inflicted by me,
> By me was he mangled and torn;
> I platted [sic] the thorns on His head,
> I pierced His hands and His side;
> But the blood an atonement hath made,
> And the Lamb for His murderers died.[26]

Here, as elsewhere, Wesley made much of the paradox that the suffering inflicted by sinners should ultimately bring those sinners salvation. Both responsibility and benefit could be understood individually:

> 1. Sinner behold what thou hast done!
> Exposed thy King to grief unknown,
> To anguish and disgrace:

Thy sins have cover'd Him with scorn,
Thy sins have crown'd His head with thorn,
And marr'd His heavenly face.

2. Yet in that Man deform'd for thee
The Fulness of the Godhead see,
That Man of grief and love
The Lord, thy Lord and God confess,
Who, by His blood and righteousness,
Hath bought Thy crown above.[27]

The hymn emphasizes, to the singer or reader, both that the suffering observed is "what thou hast done" and that it is suffered "for thee." As will be seen, this emphasis on individual responsibility for, and personal benefit from, Christ's sufferings is particularly important in Wesley's hymns, because it allowed him to give these sufferings particular and intense meanings for the individual singer or listener. The potential emotional force of this paradox is seen in the response of the "poor black": "What! was it for me? Did God suffer all this for so poor a creature as me?"

For Wesley, human beings could be held responsible for Christ's suffering: the hymns also contain the related idea that this suffering is inflicted by God the Father. In another description of the Passion, Wesley used the phrase "exacted is the legal pain," implying that the suffering of Christ is a necessary part of the satisfaction of God's anger.[28] While this idea occurs only occasionally in the hymns, it appears in conjunction with some of Wesley's most theologically extreme statements about the suffering of Christ. Describing Christ's refusal to drink wine just before his crucifixion:

Worldly consolations see!
Mix'd with gall the wine they give!
But who dies the death for me,
Will not the support receive
Will not lose one moment's pain;
Bears the full unlessen'd load,
Bears the rage of fiends and men,
Bears the utmost wrath of God![29]

This hymn strongly implies that to bear "the utmost wrath of God," it is necessary to suffer to the utmost, to refuse to "lose one moment's pain." Another (unpublished) hymn made the same point in even more extreme terms:

1. Jesus tastes the bitter cup,
The woe that yet remains,
Tastes, but will not drink it up
To stupify his pains:
Without comfort or support
He hangs and bears the wrath alone,
Will not cut his sufferings short,
Or lose a single groan.

2. Wonderful oeconomy
Of agonies Divine!
With a mind so calm and free
To suffer, Lord, is thine:
Jesus, lavish of thy blood,
Insatiably athirst for pain,
Thus thou shew'st thy zeal for God,
And thus thy love for man![30]

While expressions such as "Insatiably athirst for pain" may explain Wesley's decision not to publish this hymn, they clearly communicate his conviction that Jesus' suffering, not simply his death, was necessary for the satisfaction of God's wrath. To minimize these sufferings would be to fail to bear this wrath. Jesus' decision to bear these sufferings, as part of his atoning work, demonstrates both his "zeal for God" and his "love for man." These hymns emphasize that Jesus suffered deliberately and willingly in obedience to God the Father.

Wesley's hymns, then, reveal his understanding of Christ's suffering as a necessary element of the atonement. By suffering as Adam and his descendants were cursed to suffer, Christ bore Adam's penalty on behalf of all humanity. By suffering under God's justice, Christ satisfied his "utmost" wrath. These hymns thus introduce two notions about suffering that recur throughout Wesley's work. The first is the inevitability of human suffering in this life. For Wesley, the fall of Adam meant that all human beings suffer. As these verses suggest, such suffering is experienced in daily life, through the hard toil for "embitter'd bread"; in the experience of personal sinfulness or a "barren soul"; in the awareness of "death's sentence" and, ultimately, in the misery of hell. The primary meanings of human suffering are therefore to do with "sin and chastisement."

This understanding of human suffering was also communicated through John Wesley's sermons. John taught that suffering was God's judgment on sin: if God was to remain just, he must punish the crime of rebellion against him. In giving people free will, God allowed them the freedom to sin and suffering was the inevitable result of their exercise of this freedom.[31] According to John, God's judgment was expressed not just in the direct consequences of sinful human actions but also through the created world. For example, in the preface to his book of home remedies, *Primitive Physick*, John wrote that, prior to the sin of Adam and Eve, "heaven and earth and all the hosts of them were mild, benign, and friendly to human nature."[32] Since the entry of sin into the world, however, all of creation expressed God's judgment on sin:

> The seeds of weakness and pain, of sickness and death, are now lodged in our inmost substance; whence a thousand disorders continually spring, even without the aid of external violence. And how is the number of these increased by every thing round about us! The heavens, the earth, and all things contained therein, conspire to punish the rebels against their Creator. The sun and moon shed unwholesome influences from above; the earth exhales poisonous damps from beneath; the beasts of the field, the birds of the air, the fishes of the sea, are in a state of hostility.[33]

While God brings about this "conspiracy" of creation against humanity, he does so in response to the rebellion of human beings. Human beings are therefore ultimately responsible for the suffering that results. This same understanding can be seen in Charles's sermon on "The Cause and Cure of Earthquakes," in which he used biblical passages to argue that earthquakes are the direct judgment of God against human sinfulness. Charles distinguished between the "author," the "moral cause" and the "natural cause" of earthquakes: "God is himself the author, and sin the *moral* cause, of earthquakes (whatever the natural cause may be)."[34]

The second central notion regarding suffering that emerges from these hymns is that suffering is the means by which Christ rescues humanity from this fate: "He suffers in my stead." Christ's victory over suffering results in the ultimate end of suffering for his people, by making possible their entry into heaven. Thus while the suffering of Christ is also a matter of judgment, in which Christ bears the judgment due to sinful humanity, his sufferings are also imbued with other, more positive meanings, to do with submission to God and love for humanity. This theological context had significance for the ways in which early Methodists responded to both the suffering of Christ and their own suffering.

Suffering and Spiritual Transformation

Identifying this theological framework within Wesley's hymns is, however, only one part of the task of exploring Wesley's construction of the meaning and power of Christ's suffering. If, as I have argued, Wesley's hymns are best understood as spiritual tools, designed to shape the individual life toward spiritual ends, then it is important to consider what part Christ's suffering plays in the process of spiritual transformation. What power did Wesley understand Christ's suffering to have in the individual's life? This question can be answered by considering how Christ's suffering is constructed in Wesley's verse.

One of Wesley's lengthiest explorations of the suffering and death of Christ was in an early work titled "A Passion Hymn" (see Hymn 1). While this hymn is a more extended treatment of the Passion than most of Wesley's hymns, it provides an excellent example of the basic pattern that most of these works follow in considering Christ's suffering. It opens with a call to "behold" the suffering Jesus:

> 1. Ye that pass by, behold the Man!
> The Man of Griefs, condemn'd for you!
> The Lamb of God, for sinners slain,
> Weeping to Calvary pursue.
>
> 2. See how His back the scourges tear,
> While to the bloody pillar bound!
> The ploughers make long furrows there,
> Till all His body is one wound.

Readers or singers of the hymn are called upon to stop, to pay attention to the spectacle of Christ's pain, and visually to follow him to the cross. As the hymn twice affirms, this is the suffering of a "Man," and thus accessible to human empathy. The sensation of seeing is carefully evoked by the detailed naming of Christ's body – face, limbs, back, temples, hands, feet, side and brow – and the description of how each part suffers. The description emphasizes the passivity of his body, as it is spat upon, whipped, stretched, torn, fastened and exposed. In case our attention falters, we are reminded throughout the hymn to continue watching by the insertion of exhortations to "see" (verse two) or "see there!" (verse nine). These first verses evoke the sight of a body helplessly suffering.

Wesley's meticulous description evokes a vivid picture of human suffering, which in itself functions to produce a powerful emotional response. This response is shaped, however, by his repeated statement of the theological meanings of Christ's suffering. The hymn communicates Wesley's understanding of the meaning of the crucifixion both explicitly and more subtly in these verses. The first states clearly that the death to be witnessed is "for sinners" and this message is reinforced throughout the hymn. The initial call to "behold" in verse one uses the language of Lamentations: "Is it nothing to you, all ye that pass by? Behold and see if there be any sorrow like unto my sorrow, which is done unto me, wherewith the Lord hath afflicted me in the day of his fierce anger."[35] This lament for Jerusalem, interpreted by the Methodists as a prophetic description of Christ's crucifixion, was a favorite text for Wesley's evangelistic sermons.[36] By referring to it, Wesley hinted that the suffering to be witnessed is propitiatory, inflicted by God. This is reinforced by biblical imagery in the same verse: Jesus is the sacrificial "Lamb of God." Wesley also used biblical language in his description of the scourging. Here he employed an image from Psalm 129, from a verse again given prophetic significance by the Methodists: "The plowers plowed upon my back: they made long their furrows."[37]

By placing his description of physical suffering firmly within this theological and scriptural context, Wesley encouraged a particular emotional response. The emphasis on substitutionary atonement reminds the reader or singer that Christ's suffering was undeserved, voluntary and "for you!" That Jesus is innocent intensifies the reader's pity for him; that his death is for sinners encourages responses of gratitude and guilt.

The poem's suggestion of other contrasts and paradoxes also directs the reader's emotional response. In this description, Wesley was particularly concerned with contrasts between weakness and power, passivity and aggression. Verses three to five contrast the desecration of Jesus' face by the mob with the honor it receives from prophets and angels; the meekness and silence of Jesus with the insults and aggression of the mob; the innocence of Jesus with the rage and hate of the mob. Verse ten establishes the paradox of Jesus' suffering: "The'Immortal hangs His languid brow,/ The'Almighty faints beneath His load!" By contrasting Christ's identity as omnipotent God with his voluntary weakness and humble passivity in suffering, Wesley emphasized the sacrifice involved in this suffering. The liberal use of exclamation marks, here and throughout this description, suggest that amazement is the appropriate response to this sacrifice.

Wesley also communicated his understanding of the crucifixion with the use of images with particular significance within Methodist discourse. In verse nine, the "hands extended wide" signify the welcoming love of God; the "fountain gushing from His side" compares the blood of Jesus to a fountain that cleanses from sin.[38] While the sight of human arms stretched in crucifixion or the sight of blood gushing from wounds might be expected simply to horrify, Wesley's construction of these sights, as communicating welcoming love and mercy, evokes intimacy and gratitude as well.

The first verses of this hymn, then, establish a picture of Christ's suffering that functions to evoke emotions of profound pity, intimacy, gratitude and amazement in the reader or singer. Early in the hymn, responsibility for his suffering is established with the anonymous original actors: "they" are said to "whip," "stretch," "tear," "fasten" and "expose" Jesus. In verse eleven, however, there is a sharp twist in perspective. Through Wesley's characteristic use of the first person, the reader or singer is brought into the action as the one responsible for this suffering. This fact is reiterated in three emphatic statements:

I fill'd His soul with pangs unknown;
I caused those mortal groans and cries,
I kill'd the Father's only Son.

The full weight of the emotional response evoked by Wesley's careful description of suffering is brought to bear upon "me," making the viewer responsible (through his or her sins) for all the suffering of Jesus. Wesley established a powerful causal link between the viewer and the viewed: a linkage intellectually justified within the theological framework that the hymn reinforces, but emotionally established by the literary device of bringing the viewer into the narrative at this point.

Through the evocation of the physical presence of Jesus' battered body, and also by the drawing of this causal link that makes us, as readers or singers, responsible for what we see, in verse twelve we are imaginatively positioned close to the suffering Jesus, as part of the crowd at the foot of the cross. As this was not simply an imaginative exercise for Wesley, but also a spiritual one, the final verses are a prayer made from this position of intimacy. The content of this prayer is perhaps surprising: having established the reader's personal guilt, the hymn might be expected immediately to emphasize repentance, the renouncing of sin. Instead, verses twelve and thirteen are a prayer to feel, to "sympathise" with and to "share" in the suffering that is seen:

12. O Thou dear suffering Son of God,
How doth Thy heart to sinner's move!
Help me to catch Thy precious blood,
Help me to taste Thy dying love.

13. Give me to feel Thy agonies,
One drop of Thy sad cup afford:
I fain with Thee would sympathise,
And share the sufferings of my Lord.

Such empathetic feeling is paralleled in these verses with personal comprehension and appropriation of Christ's death, expressed as "catch[ing]" and "tast[ing]." Verses fourteen and following emphasize the need for the inward change of heart that is repentance and self-renunciation. This change is described as comparable to the earthquake that followed the crucifixion. It is the sight of the suffering Christ, and the emotional response that this sight compels, that is powerful enough to produce the inner quaking, convulsion and shakings that are necessary for this transformation.

The basic elements of this hymn, with its evocation of the sight of the suffering Christ, its explanation of this suffering in theological terms that emphasize its relevance to "me" and its urging of empathetic sorrow for the purposes of personal transformation appear in hymn after hymn that Wesley wrote. Many of these elements can be seen in Wesley's account of the "poor black" in Newgate. Wesley recorded that in his preaching he described "the sufferings of the Son of God, his sorrows, agony, & death." He assured the "poor black" that Jesus came to save "him in particular" and the man was deeply emotionally affected, leading to spiritual change. The hymn that the condemned men sang together reinforced the idea of reflecting on the sight of Christ's sufferings for spiritual benefit.

These elements can also be seen in many of the experiences of Methodists who wrote or spoke to the Wesley brothers. For example, on 19 May 1740, a Mrs. Margaret Austin of London wrote to Charles Wesley to describe her conversion. After hearing both George Whitefield and John Wesley on earlier occasions, she had attended a meeting in Wapping where Charles was speaking. "I heard you, sir," she wrote, "and there I plainly saw my Saviour bleeding on the cross, and the soldiers piercing his precious side, and the blood falling to the ground. Oh, thought I, that I had but one drop of that blood to wash away my sins."[39] Speaking to her earlier, Charles had recorded her experience in his journal in similar words: "I was justified the first Friday you were at Wapping, with those many others; saw my Saviour bringing me a pardon written in his blood."[40] The experience that Mrs. Austin and Charles Wesley recorded – of seeing the suffering Christ – is one that is repeated in many of the testimonies written by the Methodists who corresponded with John and Charles Wesley. These men and women often described transformative spiritual experiences in terms of a profound response to the sight of Christ's suffering.[41] Why did these elements combine for Methodists in such meaningful and powerful ways? To begin to answer this question, it is necessary to consider more closely the way in which Wesley constructs the relationship between the elements of sight, suffering and empathetic sorrow, as well as the cultural and religious conventions that Wesley draws upon in this construction.

Sight and Sorrow

Wesley's poetical emphasis on Christ's suffering was not, of course, original. It was part of a long tradition of Passion poetry in England, which flowered in the late medieval period, and survived after the Reformation in the works of poets such as Herbert and Herrick.[42] In the context of the evangelical revivals, Passion devotion reappeared in the form of hymns, influenced by German pietist hymn-writers who focused on Christ's sufferings.[43] Passion devotion had initially developed as part of the "affective" tradition in late medieval Christianity, which emphasized intimacy with Christ through devotion and reflection.[44] Like Methodism, this tradition placed great value on experience, on an emotional apprehension of spiritual realities.

The depiction of Christ's sufferings in Wesley's hymns is similar in many ways to late medieval depictions of the Passion, which encouraged an "understanding of the Passion as passive suffering by a loving victim by directing the devotee's attention to Christ's 'bitter sufferings' and the moment of his death."[45] Similarly, as "A Passion Hymn" suggests, many of Wesley's hymns on Christ's death take much of their emotional power from descriptions of his "bitter sufferings." Wesley used a broad range of phrases to communicate Christ's physical afflictions, many of which he used repeatedly. For example, he wrote of Christ's "mangled body torn," his "bleeding feet," his "visage marr'd with tears and blood," his "bloody sweat."[46] Elsewhere he described the instruments of Christ's suffering, such as "The thorns His temples tear"; "those nails into His body driven"; and "the whips" that tore his body.[47] As is also demonstrated by "A Passion Hymn," Wesley constructed these depictions of Christ's suffering to emphasize Christ's love, innocence and passivity. Verses from another of Wesley's hymns clearly communicate this view of Christ's sufferings:

> 13. Yes, Lord, with joy, and grief and love
> I now behold Thy face,
> My God descended from above
> To suffer in my place.
>
> 14. Thy visage marr'd with tears and blood,
> Mine eyes of faith survey,
> As when on yonder cross my God
> A bleeding Victim lay.
>
> 15. Torn with whips, and nails, and spear
> Thy sacred body was;
> O might it now to all appear
> As hanging on the cross![48]

This typical description of Christ as sacrificial "Victim" called for a response of pity and gratitude, of "joy and grief and love." Wesley's hymns provided a spiritual tool for the Methodist faithful to reflect on such depictions, and to respond in this way. In doing so, they conformed to many of the conventions of the genre of Passion devotion. These hymns are distinctive, however, in their construction, and exploration of the relationship between sight, feeling and spiritual change, particularly in the explicit emphasis given to the power of sight.

This relationship can be further analyzed in another of Wesley's hymns that explore Christ's suffering, the second hymn in a series he wrote "For Believers" (see Hymn 2). Although this hymn does not begin by considering Christ's suffering, in verse four our visual attention is again directed to the physical suffering of Christ: his wounds, his bleeding, the piercing of his hands, feet and side. Christ bows his head, he spreads his arms, his blood streams. Again, the hymn provides a theological interpretation of this suffering, with references to "the Lamb" and the clear statement that Christ "suffers in the sinner's stead." Here Wesley provided a more explicit explanation of the meanings communicated by Christ's physical pain: In verse five his arms are spread "to take me in," his blood streams "to purge my sin." This hymn is also more directive than "A Passion Hymn," as from the beginning the reader or singer is allocated the appropriate emotional response to this sight, through first-person responses interjected throughout the narrative.

The description of Christ's suffering is, however, only one event in a narrative of spiritual transformation. Verses one to three describe in great detail the evil of the singer's heart: "self-hardened" even to God's wrath and judgments. Where plagues, wrath and fear are impotent to bring about change, the love expressed in Christ's suffering is able to prevail. The sight of the cross is therefore presented to "try" the hard-hearted one. This language of judgment and rebellion, of trial and defiance, is clearly suggestive of the courtroom. That this is a trial by ordeal is made clear immediately: "Ah! who that piteous sight can bear!" The eight exclamation marks in this description of Christ's suffering suggest that the sight is indeed intensely confronting. The viewer resists for a time, but ultimately the sight overpowers, bringing about the yielding and the breaking of the heart, its "softening" and "melting."

This narrative illustrates Wesley's understanding of the relationship between the emotions and the spiritual self. Here, as elsewhere, the human heart is naturally hard: Wesley regularly described it as "stony," "flinty" or "stubborn."[49] The use of the metaphor of hard-heartedness, with its double meaning of sinful obstinacy and emotional insensitivity, demonstrates again how tightly the emotional and the spiritual are linked in Wesley's thought. The process of inner submission through which he leads the believer in this hymn is explicitly a process of emotional change: it climaxes with a description of what "I feel." The hymn produces this emotional effect: verse four describes the suffering of Christ, and then verse five emphasizes in almost every line that this suffering is for "my" benefit. The combination of pity at this suffering, with the personal recognition that this suffering is done out of love for "me," produces the profound emotional response Wesley described.

Wesley repeatedly described the spiritual change that results from seeing Christ's suffering in terms of emotion, and he repeatedly used similar techniques to produce this change, as in a verse from a hymn from a series of "Hymns for Love":

2. O might I look and mourn
O'er my Redeemer slain,
And never more to sin return,
Or pierce my Lord again!
Repentance deep and true,
Thou slaughter'd Lamb impart,
As crucified appear in view,
And break this stubborn heart.[50]

Mourning at the sight of Christ's suffering is here equivalent to repentance for one's sins, just as in "For Believers" the shedding of tears is the sign of submission to God's love. This mourning is caused both by pity at the suffering seen, and recognition that "I," the singer or reader of this hymn, am responsible for it. This produces a response of guilt and penitence.

The two elements of description of Christ's sufferings and affirmation that these sufferings are "for me" or "by me" are repeatedly tied together to produce emotional responses dominated by guilt or gratitude respectively. This is demonstrated in a hymn on Luke 23: 28.

1. Our hearts for Thee will nought avail
Unless we Lord our sins bewail,
The cause of all Thy pain,
Unless our rocky hearts be rent
In vain Thou bear'st our punishment,
And shedd'st Thy blood in vain.

2. But O, Thy blood the sorrow buys,
Thy blood the contrite grace supplies,
And melts my heart of stone:
Struck by Thy death with anguish deep,
Prostrate before Thy cross I weep,
And now myself bemoan.

3. Long as Thy mangled form appears,
I lie dissolved in gracious tears
Of love's soft sympathy:
And here I would through life remain,
And of these cruel sins complain
Which nail'd Thee to that tree.[51]

This hymn repeats the idea that an emotional response – bewailing, weeping and anguish – is necessary for Christ's death to be spiritually effective. Verse three makes it clear that this will happen when the believer sees Christ's "mangled form" and recognizes his or her own responsibility for this death. Regular exposure to hymns such as these must surely have reinforced Methodist expectations that what was needed for spiritual transformation was not mere intellectual conviction, but the overwhelming emotional response that a vision of Christ's suffering would produce.

Methodist conversion narratives echo Wesley's portrayal of the process of spiritual change as one in which a "stony" heart was powerfully overwhelmed by God.[52] These narratives describe a lengthy process of striving and struggling toward the new birth, in cycles of hope and despair, until a final breakthrough was achieved. Describing his wife's conversion, one man informed Wesley: "She laboured under the burden of her sins for near two years before she found deliverance."[53] Charles Wesley himself taught that such a struggle was a normal element in the process of conversion.[54] George Story, a Methodist preacher, wrote of his conversion,

> Attending to the experiences of the people, I observed that almost all of them, during the time of conviction, were exercised with horrible fears and terrors; and thence I concluded it was necessary I should have the same. I therefore used every method to bring myself under dreadful apprehensions, hoping this would break my stubborn heart.[55]

After failing to produce such "dreadful apprehensions" in himself, Story realized that he was wrong to presume how God would work. Instead of a violent upheaval, "the softening power of grace descended, and removed the stony heart."[56] While Story's experience is evidence that "dreadful apprehensions" were not essential, his observation that "almost all" converts went through this time of trial suggests that it was the norm.

This understanding of the conversion experience owed much to European pietism, which had emphasized the importance of the *Busskampf*, or "inward penitential struggle," before the new birth was received.[57] This model of the conversion process relied on an understanding of the self as deeply sinful and resistant to change. Disagreement over the necessity of the *Busskampf* was central to the Wesleys' split from the Moravians, and the differences between the two movements in this regard illuminate their respective portrayals of the suffering of Christ. Initially, the Wesleys had learned their model of conversion, including its emphasis on the *Busskampf*, from the Moravians. Under the leadership of Zinzendorf, however, the Moravians moved away from belief in the necessity of the *Busskampf*.[58] Instead, they emphasized the importance of a passive waiting for the new birth, during which the individual meditated deeply on the sufferings of Christ. Zinzendorf encouraged a devotion to the wounds of Christ, in particular the "side-hole" where Christ had been pierced with a spear. Moravian conversion narratives reflected the language of Moravian hymns that described living in these wounds:

> O precious Side-hole's cavity
> I want to spend my life in thee...
> There in one Side-hole's joy divine,
> I'll spend all future Days of mine.[59]

Such hymns encouraged the passive adoration of Christ's suffering; Moravians spoke of resting in, abiding in or drinking from his wounds.[60]

Neither Methodist conversion narratives nor Wesley's hymns display the insistent, detailed focus on Christ's corporeal suffering that appears in Moravian conversion narratives and hymns.[61] Wesley's hymns do, however, point to the importance of Christ's suffering in Methodist spirituality. Christ's suffering features in these hymns in ways that reflect Methodist understandings of conversion, as the sight of the Passion is described as a shocking, even violent experience. In the hymn "For Believers," the sight of Christ's suffering is a confronting ordeal, by which the believer is "constrain'd" to "yield." This forceful language is typical of Wesley's descriptions of the effect of seeing Jesus' suffering. Elsewhere the sight of Jesus' suffering is portrayed as able to "meeken," "force," "seize," "constrain," "conquer" and "blast" the viewer.[62] Wesley described the one exposed to this sight, as "humbled," "prostrate," "o'erwhelmed," "compell'd" and "subdued."[63] Such descriptions reflect the Methodist conviction that spiritual transformation was a demanding process, which required the forceful overthrowing of a stubbornly sinful will.

Wesley's portrayal of spiritual change in these terms relied on a fundamental association between the experience of sight and a powerful emotional or spiritual response. His conviction of the significance of sight was made even more explicit in a short hymn on the crucifixion:

> Who see must surely feel
> That piteous spectacle!
> Stone to flesh the sight doth turn!
> Yes I share the dying smart,
> Now I look on Thee and mourn,
> Now I give Thee all my heart.[64]

Wesley's neat reversal of the mythic idea of the sight that turns the viewer to stone demonstrates how powerful he understood this sight to be. His conviction that the sight of suffering *must* produce an intense reaction was central to his construction of Christ's suffering. This conviction, that to see is to feel, resonated powerfully with cultural trends within eighteenth-century England. This broader resonance explains something of the power of the idea of the sight of Christ's sufferings within Methodist culture.

The Culture of Sensibility

As a number of historians have suggested, eighteenth-century English culture increasingly emphasized the value of "a new set of attitudes and emotional conventions at the heart of which was a sympathetic concern for the pain and suffering of other sentient beings."[65] The value of sympathy was explored in a wide variety of texts and contexts, along with a number of related concepts such as "sentiment," "sensibility," "pity" and "benevolence." These terms are at times difficult to distinguish from one another in their eighteenth-century usage, but they all relate to the imaginative and compassionate awareness of another's feelings. Brycchan Carey has argued for the central importance within this discourse of the "relationship between sensibility, the capacity to feel, and sympathy, the capacity to imagine another's feelings as one's own."[66] In 1755 Samuel Johnson's *Dictionary* defined sympathy as "mutual sensibility."[67] The eighteenth-century "culture of sensibility" therefore valued both the ability to feel deeply and the ability to feel deeply for others.

At a philosophical level, arguments for the value of sympathy can be seen as an attempt to develop an ethical system on the basis of the empiricist claim that true knowledge comes from experience. An ethical system of this kind was particularly attractive to the growing middle class because it allowed them to achieve gentility based on a refined "sensibility" rather than noble birth or an aristocratic code of honor.[68] This emphasis on sympathy encouraged a concern for the pain and suffering of others that was evoked in campaigns for moral reform including, later in the century, the campaign for the abolition of the slave trade. The social and economic causes of this growing emphasis on empathetic compassion, and its relationship to humanitarian reform, have been debated at length.[69] The relevance of this shift to Methodism will be discussed in more detail in the following chapters.

In relation to Wesley's poetic treatment of the suffering of Christ, however, it is significant that this "culture of sensibility" included an emphasis on the emotional power of sight. Randall McGowen argues that eighteenth-century debates over public execution increasingly reflected the conviction that "[t]he eye was simply a channel for feeling."[70] To *see* suffering, such a conviction suggested, was to *feel* suffering in empathy. Exploring the connection between the senses and sympathy in detail in *The Theory of Moral Sentiments* (1759), Adam Smith concluded that the sight of suffering did not produce sympathy by itself; rather, the viewer's imaginative response produced sympathy. Smith argued that when confronted with a person in pain, we imagine ourselves undergoing the same experience. In so doing, "we enter as it was into his body, and become in some measure the same person with him, and thence form some idea of his sensations…" When this imaginative identification occurs, Smith argued, the agonies of the other person "begin at last to affect us, and then we tremble and shudder at the thought of what he feels."[71]

Smith's use of the words "tremble" and "shudder" indicates his expectation that the sight of another's suffering would powerfully, even violently, affect the empathetic viewer. As in Wesley's hymns, this could be so powerful as to be unbearable. One reformer wrote of public executions: "the bosom of humanity will heave in agony at the idea, the eye of religion will turn with horror from the spectacle."[72] Smith's argument also suggests that an empathetic response to the sight of suffering gave rise to a particularly meaningful understanding of the suffering perceived. By becoming "in some measure the same person" with the sufferer, his agonies "are thus brought home" to the viewer. To see was to feel. But in the case of suffering, it was also to understand.

Wesley's hymns clearly resonated with these convictions. Within the "culture of sympathy," it was meaningful to suggest that the sight of Christ's suffering must produce intense empathetic distress in the viewer. This was powerful to effect spiritual change because it allowed true understanding of Christ's suffering, and of the undeserved love and sacrifice that this suffering represented. This in turn would bring about the appropriate responses of repentance, love and gratitude. This process is described in a hymn reflecting on the doubt experienced by Thomas the disciple, where the language of sight, feeling and knowledge is used almost interchangeably.

1. Open mine eyes of faith to see
Thy hands and feet transfix'd and torn,
So shall I know that Thou art He
Who hast my sins and sorrows borne,
The Man that on the mountain bled,
And rose my Surety from the dead.

2. O could I now behold my Lord,
Discern and touch the Crucified,
Adore the true immortal Word,
And thrust my hand into Thy side,
And feel that Thou my Saviour art;
Whose blood is sprinkled on my heart![73]

While this hymn also expresses a desire to touch the crucified Christ (following the original account of Thomas's experience of touching Christ's wounds), here, and elsewhere in Wesley's hymns, sight was the pre-eminent sense of perception and feeling.

Wesley repeatedly contended that the relationship between sight and spiritual transformation was so significant that, without the sight of Jesus' suffering, such change was not possible. In Hymn VI from the series of "Hymns for Love," Wesley again explored the hard-heartedness of the believer and begs for the experience of true repentance and love. After a description of the believer's inability to change, the hymn continues:

3. Appear as crucified for me,
The purchase of Thy blood;
To get Thyself the victory,
Come, O my Lord, my God;
To make Thy depths of mercy known
Thy Spirit now impart,
And break by Thy expiring groan,
And take my broken heart.

4. It must, alas! continue whole
Till I my Saviour see,
As pouring out His spotless soul,
As dying on the tree:
That piteous spectacle alone
My flinty heart can move,
And turn to flesh the soften'd stone,
And melt me into love.

5. Come then, Thou slaughter'd Lamb Divine,
Thy bleeding wounds display,
And seize today this heart of mine
While it is call'd to-day:
A time to Thee I would not set,
Yet at Thy cross I bow,
Restless, resign'd, Thy coming wait,
And long to meet Thee now.[74]

At the heart of this hymn is a call to Christ to provide the supplicant with a vision of his crucified body. Unless this happens, the hymn affirms, the believer's heart cannot be transformed. The hymn describes the sufferings of Christ only in shorthand, as "bleeding wounds," or his "dying on the tree." Nonetheless, the sight of these sufferings is presented as uniquely transformative, and even the thought of them is able to produce the restless longing with which the hymn concludes. This hymn, and others like it, associates a deep longing for spiritual transformation with a longing for the sight of Christ's suffering self.

I have suggested that Wesley's emphasis on the sight of Christ's suffering as a basis for inner transformation drew on both the Christian tradition of Passion devotion as well as eighteenth-century convictions about the relationship between sight and feeling. Yet when Wesley wrote of "seeing" the suffering of Christ, he was clearly not speaking of physical sight, or necessarily of an actual vision. Rather the idea of sight, with all its cultural power, was being evoked for emotional and spiritual purposes. Unlike medieval Passion texts, Wesley's hymns did not interact with a wide range of visual depictions of Christ's suffering, nor with a culture of pilgrimage and relics.[75] Evangelical culture as a whole emphasized the spiritual value of hearing (the word of God) rather than seeing (which could encourage idolatry).[76] The hymns considered here assume the power and value of the imagination in producing spiritual experiences, rather than that of actual images or objects. The imaginative quality of the sight that Wesley affirms can be seen by considering a number of Wesley's "Hymns on the Lord's Supper."

In this collection, Wesley repeatedly presented the bread and wine of communion as visual prompts for reflection on Christ's suffering. "Hymn II" from this series presents a meditative cycle that begins and ends with the communion bread, presumably physically present before the reader or singer (Hymn 3). This hymn begins with Wesley's typical evocation of sight: "In this expressive bread I see,/ The wheat by man cut down for me." The physical suffering of Christ is described, its theological significance pointed out, and once again the hymn indicates that this suffering is "for me." Perhaps because of the parallels being drawn with the bread, the active role of God the Father in inflicting this suffering is described in more explicit and detailed terms than usual. Christ is victim of both "man and God." The aim of this hymn seems to be to prepare for communion and so the hymn ends by pointing to the bread (which in Wesley's theology is itself a source of spiritual change) rather than describing spiritual change.

While Wesley's description of the bread may suggest that he placed a spiritual value on actually looking at the bread, a closer examination makes clear his preference for "inner" rather than "outer" sight. He wrote that in the bread it was possible to "see" certain things – the beating and bruising of the wheat, the drying and roasting of the bread – that symbolize the suffering of Christ. In reality, these processes cannot be seen in the bread because the bread is only their result. Ultimately, the bread acts as a prompt to imagining Christ's suffering, not because of any visual resemblance, but because of a theological connection. For Wesley the bread actually represented Christ's body: "my Lord is here become/ The Bread of Life to me." Understanding this connection requires a different kind of seeing, as Wesley made explicit in "Hymn CXL" of the series: "Now with faith's interior eye/ Behold Him stand as slaughter'd there."[77] "Faith's interior eye" sees more powerfully than the physical eye. Wesley himself recorded such an experience in the context of the Lord's Supper, writing in his journal:

> I left it to Christ, whether, or in what measure, he would please to manifest himself to me, in this breaking of bread. I had no particular attention to the prayers: but in the prayer of consecration I saw, by the eye of faith, or rather, had a glimpse of, Christ's broken, mangled body, as taking [sic] down from the cross.[78]

While Wesley uses the language of sight, in his hymns he ultimately devalues the potential of physical sight in favor of an interior, imaginative, spiritual seeing. Wesley's repeated call to "see" is a call to visualize, and Methodists singing Wesley's hymns would continually rehearse the experience of visualizing the suffering of Christ.

Charles Wesley's emphasis on the potential benefits of seeing with "faith's interior eye" was not original. As has been mentioned, John Wesley argued for a category of spiritual senses, contending that:

> It is necessary that you have *the hearing ear*, and the *seeing eye*, emphatically so called; that you have a new class of senses opened in your soul, not depending on organs of flesh and blood, to be "the *evidence* of things not seen" as your bodily senses are of visible things, to be the avenues to the invisible world, to discern spiritual objects."[79]

If John spoke of "a new class of senses," to explain what faith perceived, Charles's hymns trained these senses, particularly sight, to work in particular ways. Spiritual sight, in Charles's hymns, functioned in ways that fitted with his culture's understanding of how "the outward eye" worked.

The Power of the Passion

Throughout Charles Wesley's hymns, the sufferings of Christ are endowed with profound meaning and great power. The theological significance that the hymns give to these sufferings places them, with Christ's death, at the center of the atonement. Because these sufferings are substitutionary, they point to human suffering as being primarily a matter of God's judgment. Human suffering is directly or indirectly the result of human sin. By suffering in the place of sinners, however, Christ rescues human beings from this judgment. In doing so, he invests suffering with new, redemptive meanings.

Beyond these theological meanings, however, the hymns credit Christ's Passion with power to transform the human heart through an encounter, preferably visual. That such encounters were part of Methodist culture is seen in the experience of Margaret Austin and those other Methodists who recorded their own transformative experiences of seeing Christ's suffering, precisely those experiences that Wesley's hymns were intended to evoke, rehearse and reinforce. John Wesley recorded in his journal the testimony of a young Methodist woman, who told him:

> On Friday, the 4th of last March, I was sitting in the house while one read the Passion Hymn. I had always before thought myself good enough, having constantly gone to church and said my prayers, nor had I ever heard any of the Methodist preachers. On a sudden I saw my Saviour on the cross as plain as if it had been with my bodily eyes; and I felt it was *my* sins for which He died. I cried out and had no strength left in me. Whether my eyes were open or shut, He was still before me hanging on the cross; and I could do nothing but weep and mourn day and night.[80]

For this young woman, the words of Charles's "Passion Hymn" triggered an experience of profound and transformative power.[81]

Many Methodists did not record visual experiences of this kind, but the broader pattern of a transformative encounter with the love of Christ, expressed in his sufferings, is repeated throughout Methodist writings. On 28 November 1746, Wesley described his attendance at a Methodist meeting in Newcastle: "I set before their eyes Christ crucified, and crying from the cross, 'Is it nothing to you, all ye that pass by?' The rocks were melted into gracious tears."[82] Wesley's understanding of spiritual change and maturity required the constant "melting" of the hard human heart in response to God's love as demonstrated by "Christ crucified." The hymns provided a powerful tool for this purpose: they evoked Christ's suffering in ways that explicitly encouraged an intensely emotional response. In so doing, they gave the suffering of Christ a central place in Methodist spirituality. As the following chapter will demonstrate, this had profound significance for Wesley's construction of the Christian life.

[Hymn 1]
A Passion Hymn

1. Ye that pass by, behold the Man!
The Man of Griefs, condemn'd for you!
The Lamb of God, for sinners slain,
Weeping to Calvary pursue.

2. See how His back the scourges tear,
While to the bloody pillar bound!
The ploughers make long furrows there,
Till all His body is one wound.

3. The abjects spit upon that face
Which prophets wished in vain to see,
On which the angels loved to gaze,
Pleased with His milder majesty.

4. Adored by angels, mock'd by men,
Speechless the form of guilt He wears;
Reviled, He answers not again,
But meekly all their insults bears.

5. Nor can He thus their hate assuage;
His innocence, to death pursued,
Most fully glut their utmost rage:
Hark! how they clamour for His blood!
.....

8. His sacred limbs they stretch, they tear,
With nails they fasten to the wood;
His sacred limbs – exposed, and bare,
Or only cover'd with His blood.

9. See there! His temples crown'd with thorns!
His bleeding hands extended wide,
His streaming feet, transfixt and torn!
The fountain gushing from His side!

10. Where is the King of Glory now?
The everlasting Son of God!
The'Immortal hangs His languid brow,
The'Almighty faints beneath His load!

11. Beneath *my* load He faints and dies:
I fill'd His soul with pangs unknown;
I caused those mortal groans and cries,
I kill'd the Father's only Son.

12. O Thou dear suffering Son of God,
How doth Thy heart to sinner's move!
Help me to catch Thy precious blood,
Help me to taste Thy dying love.

13. Give me to feel Thy agonies,
One drop of Thy sad cup afford:
I fain with Thee would sympathise,
And share the sufferings of my Lord.

14. The earth could to her centre quake,
Convulsed, while her Creator died:
O, let my inmost nature shake,
And die with Jesus crucified!

15. At Thy last gasp the graves display'd
Their horrors to the upper skies:
O that my soul might burst the shade,
And, quicken'd by Thy death, arise.
...
18. Thy grace I surely shall receive,
Thy death hath brought the grace for me:
This is my whole desire, to live;
To live, and then to die in Thee.[83]

[Hymn 2]

Hymn II. (For Believers)

1. O what an evil, faithless heart
Have I, so ready to depart
From Thee, the living God!
Not all Thy threats, and judgments move
Till master'd by Thy stronger love,
It will not bear Thy rod.

2. The sorest plague Thou hast to send,
Nor sin itself my soul can bend,
Or bring my spirit down;
Sin makes me prouder than before,
And blinds, and hardens more and more,
Till all my heart is stone.

3. My stony heart Thy wrath defies,
And dares against Thy judgments rise,
Self-harden'd from Thy fear;
What canst Thou with Thy rebel do?
Try me by love, and in my view
With all Thy wounds appear.

4. Ah! who that piteous sight can bear!
Behold the Lamb hangs bleeding there!
There, there! on yonder tree!
Pierced are His feet, His hands, His side!
My Lamb, my Love is crucified!
O God! He dies for me!

5. For me He meekly bows His head,
He suffers in the sinner's stead,
My ruin to retrieve:
He spreads His arms to take me in,
He sheds His blood to purge my sin;
He dies that I may live.

6. O Love, by Thee constrain'd at last,
I yield, I yield; my tears flow fast,
Fast as Thy streaming blood!
Breaks at the sight my heart of stone;
I faint to hear that dying groan,
Why, O my God! My God! –

7. O God, I can hold out no more,
My heart resents Thy softening power,
My heart is melting wax;
I feel that Thou art love indeed,
Thou wilt not break the bruised reed,
Or quench the smoking flax.

8. Thou wilt not slight the feeblest grace,
This spark of love Thy breath shall raise,
And kindle to a flame;
And I, who taste how good Thou art,
Shall shortly love with all my heart
My lovely, bleeding Lamb.[84]

[Hymn 3]
Hymn II (Hymns on the Lord's Supper)

1. In this expressive bread I see,
The wheat by man cut down for me,
And beat, and bruised, and ground:
The heavy plagues, and pains, and blows,
Which Jesus suffer'd from His foes,
Are in this emblem found.

2. The bread dried up and burnt with fire
Presents my Father's vengeful ire,
Which my Redeemer bore:

Into His bones the fire He sent,
Till all the flaming darts were spend,
And Justice ask'd no more.

3. Why hast Thou, Lord, forsook Thine own?
Alas, what evils hath He done,
That spotless Lamb of God?
Cut off, not for Himself, by me,
He bears my sins on yonder tree,
And pays my debt in blood.

4. Seized by the rage of sinful man
I see Him bound and bruised and slain;
'Tis done, the Martyr dies!
His life to ransom ours is given,
And lo! the fiercest fire of heaven
Consumes the Sacrifice.

5. He suffers both from man and God,
He bears the universal load
Of guilt and misery;
He suffers to reverse our doom;
And lo! my Lord is here become
The Bread of Life to me.[85]

Notes

1. 10 July 1738. *CWJ* 1: 17. Wesley had visited those in prison in his Oxford days, but his conversion experience and the accompanying changes in his theology meant that he now believed he should preach to the prisoners of the "new birth."

2. 12 July 1738. *CWJ* 1: 120. Peter Linebaugh identifies the "poor black" as Isaac George, a sailor from New England. Peter Linebaugh, *The London Hanged: Crime and Civil Society in the Eighteenth Century* (London: Penguin, 1991), 135–36.

3. *CWJ* 1: 122.

4. *CWJ* 1: 122–23.

5. This categorization is suggested in Alister E. McGrath, *Christian Theology: An Introduction* (Oxford: Blackwell, 1994), 341.

6. Wesley's theology of the atonement is explored in detail in John R. Tyson, "Charles Wesley's Theology of the Cross: An Examination of the Theology and Method of Charles Wesley as seen in his Doctrine of the Atonement" (PhD diss., Drew University, 1983).

7. McGrath, *Christian Theology*, 341.

8. This summary of penal substitution draws on McGrath, *Christian Theology*, 350–52; Newport, ed., *Sermons*, 62.

9. Sermon 6: Romans 3: 23–24. Newport, ed., *Sermons*, 171. Wesley quotes the same passage in Sermon 7: Romans 3: 23–25. *Sermons*, 200.

10. *SHSPHS* (1762): "Mark 15: 25." *PW* 11: 87.

11. Sermon 7: Romans 3: 23–25. Newport, ed., *Sermons*, 200.

12. In John Wesley's sermon "The Great Privilege of those that are born of God," he distinguished carefully between justification and the new birth. "God in justifying us does something for us; in begetting us again he does the work in us. The former changes our outward relation to God, so that of enemies we become children; by the latter our inmost souls are changed, so that of sinners we become saints." That which the believer sensibly experiences, therefore, is the new birth. But the new birth is a sign of justification. Albert C. Outler, ed., *Sermons I*, vol. 1, *BEW* (Nashville: Abingdon Press, 1984), 431–32.

13. 19 May 1738. *CWJ* 1: 89.

14. The experience of "receiving the atonement" is discussed in Berger, *Theology in Hymns?*, 125–29.

15. John R. Tyson, "Charles Wesley's Theology of Redemption: A Study in Structure and Method," *Wesleyan Theological Journal* 20, no. 1 (1985): 4.

16. SHSPHS (1762): "Jeremiah 8: 22." *PW* 10: 18.

17. Tyson, "Charles Wesley's Theology of Redemption," 9. As Tyson points out, this doctrine is generally credited first to Ireneaus, a second-century theologian. I have drawn on Tyson's summary of recapitulation for my explanation above.

18. Sermon 21: Luke 10: 42. Newport, ed., *Sermons*, 364.

19. Newport, ed., *Sermons*, 361.

20. *Hymns on God's Everlasting Love* (1741): "Jesus Christ, the Saviour of all men." *PW* 3: 22–23.

21. Sermon 12: Luke 18: 9–14. Newport, ed., *Sermons*, 275–76. Emphasis mine.

22. Sermon 10: John 8: 1–11. Newport, ed., *Sermons*, 253. Emphasis mine.

23. *SHSPHS* (1762): "Genesis 3: 17–19." *PW* 9: 9–10.

24. *SHSPHS* (1762): "John 19: 1." *PW* 12: 79. God's forsaking of Christ on the cross is interpreted within the same framework in "Matthew 27: 46," *PW* 12: 97–98.

25. *UP* 2: 196. (Luke 22: 44: "And his sweat was as it were great drops of blood falling down to the ground.")

26. *Sacramental Hymns* (nd): "Hymn II." *PW* 13: 260.

27. *SHSPHS* (1762): "John 14: 5 (i)." *PW* 12: 79–80.

28. *SHSPHS* (1762): "John 14: 30." *PW* 12: 100.

29. *SHSPHS* (1762): "Matthew 27: 34 (i)." *PW* 10: 427.

30. "Mark 15: 23." *UP* 2: 66.

31. See John Wesley, "On Divine Providence." Outler, ed., *Sermons II*, vol. 2, *BEW*, 534–50.

32. John Wesley, *Primitive Physic: or, An Easy and Natural Method of Curing Most Diseases*, 14th ed. (Bristol: Mr. Wesley's New Room, 2003), iii.

33. Wesley, *Primitive Physic*, iii–iv.

34. Sermon 9: Psalm 46: 8 [The Cause and Cure of Earthquakes]. Newport, ed., *Sermons*, 227. Emphasis in original.

35. Lamentations 12: 1.

36. Wesley recorded in his journal that he preached on this verse on 1 Nov. 1743, *CWJ* 1: 357; 12 Feb. 1744, *CWJ* 1: 358; 30 July 1744, *CWJ* 1: 396; 27 Nov. 1744, *CWJ* 1: 407; 8 June 1746, *CWJ* 1: 436; 28 Nov. 1746, *CWJ* 1: 456; 13 Sept. 1747, *CWJ* 1: 474.

37. Psalm 129: 3.

38. Wesley makes this explicit in the hymn "For Believers," which is discussed in detail later in this chapter.

39. Mrs. Margaret Austin to Charles Wesley, 19 May 1740. EMV 1.

40. 5 April 1740. *CWJ* 1: 207.

41. For other examples, see Elizabeth Downs to Charles Wesley, 13 Apr. 1742. EMV 53; Francis Cowper to Charles Wesley, 1741. EMV 42; Joan Webb to Charles Wesley, May 1742. EMV 136; Mary Jane Ramsey to Charles Wesley, 4 June 1740. EMV 13;

Sarah Barber to Charles Wesley, May 1740. EMV 7. See also "The Life of Thomas Olivers," in *Lives of Early Methodist Preachers, Chiefly Written by Themselves*, ed. Thomas Jackson (Stoke-on-Trent: Tentmaker Publishers, 1998), 1: 290. Also, the account of Sampson Staniforth's life in *Arminian Magazine* 6 (1783): 72, quoted in Hindmarsh, *The Evangelical Conversion Narrative*, 1.

42. See J. A. W. Bennett, *Poetry of the Passion: Studies in Twelve Centuries of English Verse* (Oxford: Clarendon Press, 1982).

43. Bennett, *Poetry of the Passion*, 168–89.

44. For discussion of this tradition see Eamon Duffy, *The Stripping of the Altars: Traditional Religion in England, c. 1400–c. 1580* (New Haven, London: Yale University Press, 1992); A. A. MacDonald, H. N. B. Ridderbos and R. M. Schlusemann, eds., *The Broken Body: Passion Devotion in Late Medieval Culture* (Groningen: Egbert Forsten, 1998).

45. Duffy, *Stripping of the Altars*, 211.

46. *PW* 1: 337, 5: 15, 5: 20, 7: 65.

47. *PW* 9: 9, 12: 86, 5: 20.

48. *HSP* (1749): "The Same. In the Work [of Charity]." *PW* 5: 19–21.

49. For example, *Hymns for Love* (nd): "Hymn VI." *PW* 8: 359–61.

50. *Hymns for Love* (nd): "Hymn VII." *PW* 8: 361.

51. *SHSPHS* (1762): "Luke 23: 28." *PW* 11: 300. Luke 23:28 – "But Jesus turning unto them said, Daughters of Jerusalem, weep not for me, but weep for yourselves, and for your children."

52. Hindmarsh, *The Evangelical Conversion Narrative*, 158.

53. "Joanna Barber's Death," Feb. 1742, EMV. Quoted in Hindmarsh, *The Evangelical Conversion Narrative*, 141.

54. Sermon 4: 1 John 3: 14. Newport, ed., *Sermons*, 133–51.

55. George Story in Mrs. Frank Stephens, ed., *Lives of the Early Methodist Preachers* (London: Horace Marshall and Son, 1903), 101.

56. Stephens, ed., *Lives of the Early Methodist Preachers*, 101.

57. Hindmarsh, *The Evangelical Conversion Narrative*, 59.

58. For the disagreements between the Wesleys and the Moravians, see Rack, *Reasonable Enthusiast*, 202–7.

59. Quoted by Thompson, *The Making of the English Working Class*, 408.

60. Hindmarsh, *The Evangelical Conversion Narrative*, 177–80. See also the discussion of Moravian devotion to the wounds as "maternal" in Mack, "Religious Dissenters in Enlightenment England," 2.

61. Hindmarsh, *The Evangelical Conversion Narrative*, 180.

62. *PW* 5: 61–62, 8: 360, 10: 255, 11: 327, 12: 86.

63. *PW* 10: 425, 11: 87, 12: 72, 12: 111.

64. *SHSPHS* (1762): "Zechariah 12: 10." *PW* 10: 122.

65. Karen Halttunen, "Humanitarianism and the Pornography of Pain in Anglo-American Culture," *The American Historical Review* 100, no. 2 (1995): 303. For other discussions of the "culture of sensibility," see Barker-Benfield, *The Culture of Sensibility*; Norman S. Fiering, "Irresistible Compassion: An Aspect of Eighteenth-Century Sympathy and Humanitarianism," *Journal of the History of Ideas* 37, no. 2 (Apr.–June 1976): 195–218; Janet Todd, *Sensibility: An Introduction* (London, New York: Methuen, 1986).

66. Brycchan Carey, "John Wesley's *Thoughts upon Slavery* and the Language of the Heart," *Bulletin of the John Rylands University Library of Manchester* 85, nos. 2 and 3 (2003): 284.

67. Carey, "John Wesley's *Thoughts upon Slavery*."

68. Paul Langford, *A Polite and Commercial People: England, 1727–1783* (Oxford: Clarendon Press, 1989), 463–65.

69. For this debate see, for example, John Ashworth, "The Relationship between Capitalism and Humanitarianism," *The American Historical Review* 92, no. 4 (1987): 813–28; Thomas L. Haskell, "Capitalism and the Origins of Humanitarian Sensibility, Part 1," *The American Historical Review* 90, no. 2 (1985): 339–61; Thomas L. Haskell, "Capitalism and the Origins of Humanitarian Sensibility, Part 2," *The American Historical Review* 90, no. 3 (1985): 547–66.

70. Randall McGowen, "The Body and Punishment in Eighteenth-Century England," *The Journal of Modern History* 59, no. 4 (1987): 673.

71. Adam Smith, *The Theory of Moral Sentiments*, ed. D. D. Raphael and A. L. Macfie (Oxford: Oxford University Press, 1976), 9.

72. Henry Dagge, *Considerations on Criminal Law* (Dublin, 1772), 226; quoted in McGowen, "The Body and Punishment," 673.

73. *SHSPHS* (1762): "Luke 24: 39". *PW* 11: 312. Luke 24: 39: "Behold my hands and my feet, that it is I myself: handle me, and see; for a spirit hath not flesh and bones, as ye see me have."

74. *Hymns for Love* (nd): "Hymn VI." *PW* 8: 359–60.

75. Duffy argues that late medieval Passion devotion was tightly linked to visual representations of Christ's suffering, which were "often conceived as channels of sacred power independent of the texts they accompanied." Duffy, *Stripping of the Altars*, 214.

76. The evangelical emphasis on "hearing" is explored in Leigh Eric Schmidt, *Hearing Things: Religion, Illusion, and the American Enlightenment* (Cambridge, Mass., and London: Harvard University Press, 2000). Schmidt argues that evangelical culture resisted the "Enlightenment" emphasis on seeing; my analysis suggests a slightly different conclusion.

77. *Hymns on the Lord's Supper* (1745): "Hymn CXL." *PW* 3: 321.

78. 25 May 1738. *CWJ* 1: 91–96.

79. John Wesley, "The Appeals to Men of Reason and Religion" in Gerald R. Cragg, ed., *Appeals to Men of Reason and Religion*, vol. 11, *BEW* (Oxford: Oxford University Press, 1975), 56–57.

80. 29 Aug. 1748. W. R. Ward and Richard P. Heitzenrater, eds., *Journals and Diaries III (1743–54)*, vol. 20, *BEW* (Nashville: Abingdon Press, 1991), 246.

81. The "Passion Hymn" also figures in an anonymous account of an execution written to Charles Wesley, in which one of the condemned men, as soon as he arrived at Tyburn, requested, "Let us sing the Passion Hymn, I love that hymn exceedingly." "Account of Executions." EMV 141.

82. 28 Nov. 1746. *CWJ* 1: 436.

83. "A Passion Hymn." *PW* 2: 70–72.

84. *HSP* (1749): "For Believers, Hymn II." *PW* 5: 2–3.

85. *Hymns on the Lord's Supper* (1745): "Hymn II." *PW* 3: 191–92.

Chapter Four

Suffering and the Christian Story

Sometime in the late 1750s, Sarah Ryan, a Methodist leader in Bristol, wrote urgently to her aging mother, who was seriously ill:

> [I]t appears we shall not see each other again on this side eternity... May the Lord bear you up. O that your hands may not hang down, nor your knees be feeble – my dear Mother look to Jesus the author till he become the finisher of your faith. Fear not, soon you shall lay this weary body down – the cross exchanges for a crown.[1]

Describing her mother's experience of illness and old age, Ryan interpreted it in terms of "the cross" and expressed her confidence that it would eventually be exchanged for "a crown." In doing so, Ryan made sense of her mother's difficulties through a narrative structure that appears repeatedly in Charles Wesley's hymns. This narrative encouraged Methodists like Ryan to understand the suffering of Christian believers through the story of Christ's suffering, to believe that trials were a "cross" that would ultimately lead to the "crown" of heavenly reward.

Wesley's hymns led Methodists to meditate upon the suffering of Christ as a source of spiritual transformation. They also encouraged Methodists to find in the story of Christ's suffering a model for their own lives and the meaning of their own sufferings. In considering the ways in which such believers might interpret their sufferings, this chapter will consider the experience of a number of early Methodist converts, including Sarah Ryan. Ryan was a controversial figure in early Methodist circles, having a pre-conversion history of sexual scandal, syphilis and a bigamous marriage. A confidant of John Wesley, she claimed to have received entire sanctification during the mid-1750s. In the autobiographical account she dictated to her companion Mary Bosanquet and in her other writings, Ryan described almost continuous experiences of intense physical, emotional and spiritual pain. Upon Ryan's death, Bosanquet commented that her life had been "as full of crosses as almost any I have ever known."[2] Ryan's writings are thus one of a number of rich sources for considering the relationship between the understandings of suffering promoted by Methodist leaders such as John and Charles Wesley, and the experience of "ordinary" believers.

Conversion and the Penitential Struggle

To understand Charles Wesley's representation of Christian suffering, it is necessary to revisit his portrayal of the experience of conversion, which established concepts of sin, holiness, personal agency and submission that were central to his construction of Christian suffering. Within early Methodism, the suffering attendant on the Christian life was often portrayed as beginning before the moment of conversion. Sarah Ryan described her state of mind prior to hearing the Methodist gospel: "my distress was very great and I knew not where to turn for help, it seemed in vain to pray. I could have no hope of mercy, nor could I discern the least ray of light amidst this terrible darkness."[3] It was only after many months in this state, close to despair, that Ryan eventually received the new birth and an assurance of sins forgiven. Her experience followed the model repeatedly described in Wesley's sermons and hymns, as well as many other conversion narratives, which presented conversion as a process requiring an initial spiritual struggle or *Busskampf*.[4] This important aspect of Methodist conversion was mentioned in the previous chapter, but its significance as an experience of suffering bears closer consideration.

In an early sermon Charles Wesley outlined this struggle very clearly.[5] He claimed that there were three classes of people: the unawakened person, entirely given over to selfish desires; the awakened or convicted person, who knew his or her own sinfulness but was powerless to change; and the person who had been born again and so delivered from the power of sin. Conversion required a progression from the first of these states to the third. The unawakened person must be confronted with the full demands of God's law and so recognize his or her own sinfulness. Wesley emphasized that God's law demanded not just outward conformity to religion, but also inner perfection of the spirit.

Wesley defined this perfection in terms of complete submission to God. He compared the external respectability of many so-called Christians to the standard implied by Christ's words: "If any man will come after me, let him deny himself, and take up his cross and follow me."

> These words demonstrate the utter impossibility of any man's becoming a Christian till he is thoroughly convinced that he is not his own, he is not the proprietor of himself, or anything he enjoys, he has no right to dispose of his goods, body, soul or any of the actions or possessions of him; and, till... he does endeavour to live, not to himself, not to pursue his own desires, not to please himself, or to suffer his own will to be any principle of action to him.[6]

When people understood God's law in these terms, recognizing that it demanded complete submission of the self to God, they would realize how deeply they had transgressed against it.

This realization, Wesley told his hearers, would be emotionally devastating. In his sermon, he described the experience of a person awakened to the reality of his or her sin, but unable to stop sinning. The imagined sinner prays, "resolves and strives, but all in vain: the more he labours, the less he prevails; the more he struggles, the faster he is bound: so that after a thousand, thousand repeated defeats he finds at last that sin is irresistible." While the awakened person would find him or herself powerless to stop sinning, Wesley exhorted those in this state not to give up striving: "You must despair before you can hope. Out of the deep must you call upon him, for it is from thence only that he will hear your voice: out of the depth of invincible sin and remorseful misery."[7] It was to those in this state of suffering, Wesley assured his listeners, that God would certainly respond with the new birth, granting forgiveness and the power to overcome sin.

Wesley's hymns encouraged a similar view of the painful struggle that faced those who recognized their own need of salvation. In the fourth of a series under the title "Groaning for Redemption," he portrayed the awakened person examining his or her soul.

2. I am the man who long have known
The strength and rage of inbred sin;
My soul is dead, my heart is stone,
A cage of birds and beasts unclean,
A den of thieves, a dire abode
Of dragons, but no house of God.

3. I dare not speak, I cannot show
The depths of Satan harbour'd there,
The horrors of infernal woe,
The black and blasphemous despair;
Who can conceive, but those that feel
Indwelling sin, indwelling hell!

4. A stranger intermeddleth not
With our inexplicable grief;
'Tis past the reach of human thought,
The torture of this unbelief,
The struggling groan, the passion loud,
The heart that says, There is no God.[8]

Significantly, the narrator is portrayed as being distressed primarily by the experience of moral uncleanness and unbelief, rather than by the consequences of sinful actions or the possibility of hell. Wesley's hymns certainly mention the threat of hell, but very few contain detailed descriptions of the sufferings that the damned would encounter there. Similarly, the consequences of sinful behavior for the individual or others are rarely mentioned. Rather, the hymns focus on an inner sense of sinfulness, which involves both an awareness of one's own moral failings and a strong sense of powerlessness to change. To Wesley, the inner self was dark and disgusting, full of unclean "beasts" and "birds." His hymns describe the "torture" of an awareness of sin in physical as well as emotional terms: as in this hymn, it typically involves struggling, weeping, groaning, fainting, laboring or an inability to speak.[9] Only those who have experienced this suffering can understand it; for the "stranger" it is "inexplicable."

The terrible pain of this experience comes not only from a consciousness of uncleanness, but also from the inability to change. In another hymn from this series, Wesley described the "anguish" of the combination of helplessness and desperate effort that would typify the person under conviction (see Hymn 1). The self is bound by sin, but struggling to be free. Wesley's description of the sinful state as an inability to "come to God" or "fear" him reinforces an understanding of sin as an inability to submit to God. This sin is like a poison that enters into the deepest part of the self, quenching hope, tempting the convicted person to suicide (the "hand of *Saul*") and inviting the just judgment of God.[10] The hymn thus encourages that "remorseful misery," to which Wesley preached God would respond. The penitent person can only hope that God will respond by transforming his or her heart in "a miracle of grace."

Wesley's poetic descriptions of this experience may seem melodramatic, but as has already been noted, many (though certainly not all) Methodists claimed to have experienced just such anguish before conversion. After hearing a Methodist preacher, Margaret Austin "was in great agonies grieving over my stony heart, and the people would pity me. But I thought I had rather they had beat me, for I deserved no pity."[11] For seventeen months she agonized, moving between extremes of hope and despair, before she finally experienced "old things passing away and all things becoming new" under Wesley's ministry. Other Methodists wrote of the lengthy distress they experienced when convinced of their sins, often feeling physical pain or being tempted to suicide.[12]

In portraying the experience of conviction in these terms, Wesley's hymns constructed the inner self of the individual in particular ways. Hindmarsh argues that evangelical preaching about sin and grace "seemed to name and call into being a new sense of interiority for… converts, a new space of moral and spiritual agency."[13] In his hymns for those convicted of sin, Wesley encouraged individuals to focus on just such an interior space, which he variously referred to as the "heart," the "soul" or the "spirit." The hymns constructed this space as initially a place of hardness and uncleanness. Sinfulness was not simply an objective state of being, but an experienced reality. Wesley's hymns described what sin *felt* like: a sense of one's inner self as stubborn and "self-harden'd," as "A cage of birds and beasts unclean,/ A den of thieves, a dire abode/ of dragons."

By emphasizing the need to struggle against this state of sinfulness, the hymns also encouraged readers or singers to focus on their own moral and spiritual agency. The hymns portrayed the "soul" or "spirit" of the unconverted person as entirely controlled by the sinful self, referred to as "the will" or "nature" or "the flesh." Before conversion, a person's spiritual power was therefore limited: the soul was "dead" and "bound"; the spirit struggled but was overcome by the flesh. Individuals were still responsible for their own state, however, and the hymns encouraged the belief that salvation would bring a new power to change, which would involve the power to submit to God rather than to sin and self.

The relationship between Christ, the self and the will can be seen in a hymn of Charles's that was published by John Wesley under the title "For Mourners brought to the Birth."

1. O my God, what must I do?
Thou alone the way canst show.
Thou canst save me in this hour;
I have neither will nor power.
God if over all thou art,
Greater than the sinner's heart,
All thy power on me be shown,
Take away the heart of stone.

2. Take away my darling sin,
Make me willing to be clean;
Make me willing to receive
All thy goodness waits to give.
Force me Lord, with all to part,
Tear these idols from my heart;
Now, thy love almighty show,
Make ev'n me a creature new.

3. Jesus, mighty to renew,
Work in me to will and do;
Turn my nature's rapid tide,
Stem the torrent of my pride;
Stop the whirlwind of my will,
Speak, and bid the sun stand still;
Now thy love almighty show,
Make ev'n me a creature new.[14]

Here the narrator prays for an experience of God's power that will overcome the sinful "nature" and create a new, believing, humble heart. The complicated place of individual agency in this process can be seen in Charles's use of the word "will." In the first verse, the narrator confesses that he or she has "neither will nor power" to believe and be saved. The second verse, therefore, is a prayer to be made "willing" to repent and receive salvation. As the third verse makes clear, however, this requires Jesus to "will and do" within the narrator. Jesus must work within the individual to "stop the whirlwind" of his or her "will." In conversion, therefore, the individual is not simply given a new ability to control him or herself. Rather, in conversion, Jesus takes control of the individual. It is the will of Jesus, working in the heart of the convert, which gives the convert a new ability to change.

Hymns such as this one created the context for a particular kind of encounter with Christ, which the previous chapter explored. A confronting experience of Christ overcame the rebelliousness of the will, melted the "stony" heart, provided assurance that the individual's moral failings had been forgiven and, as will be seen, gave the convert a new power to change. The transformative power of this experience for Methodists should not be underestimated. Repeatedly, those who wrote to Wesley described their joy, relief, love and gratitude for the change they experienced through conversion.[15] After months of anxiety and distress, Sarah Ryan experienced the forgiveness of sins while receiving the sacraments from John Wesley. "I was filled with love," she remembered, "a great change seemed to pass within me." Afterwards, she recounted "my peace and power sweetly abode and my soul did indeed walk and talk with God." [16]

Wesley himself wrote multiple hymns describing the joy of "receiving the atonement" and feeling one's sins forgiven. The Methodist preacher Mary Taft quoted one of these when she described her conversion:

> Just when I was ready to despair of the mercy of God and about to give it all up for lost, in a moment these words were applied to my heart: "Thy sins which are many are all forgiven thee." I said, yea Lord, I feel they are. My sorrow was fled; love and joy sprung up in my heart. I was ready to shout, "Come all the world, come sinner thou,/ All things in Christ are ready now."[17]

This joy reflects the experiential nature of Methodist conversion: Taft had felt herself deeply sinful and destined for hell, now she felt herself fully forgiven and heading for heaven. The terrible experience of struggling over sin meant that, for many Methodists, sin could be understood as a kind of suffering and conversion was experienced as a rescue from suffering.

Scholars strongly disagree about the social, cultural and psychological implications of conversion experiences such as Ryan's or Taft's. Methodist writings emphasized the transformative power of the experience of conversion, in relieving the terrible pressure of the struggle over sin, in bringing about a delivery from old patterns of behavior and in energizing new attitudes and activities. In Wesley's hymns, life after conversion was portrayed as conforming to a new, distinctive narrative, and his hymns provided a new language with which this experience could be described. The Christian life resembled that of Christ, in that it was experienced as a cross of suffering followed eventually by a crown of reward.

Suffering and the Christian Life

Wesley's hymns repeatedly present the sufferings and death of Christ as a pattern for the experience of Christian life. This can be seen clearly in a hymn on Hebrews 2: 10, a verse that describes Jesus as being made "perfect through sufferings" (see Hymn 2). The hymn begins with a rhetorical question prompted by this biblical assertion: "Could sufferings heighten or complete/ His full essential holiness?" The answer, of course, is no. Wesley was careful to avoid readings of this Bible verse that suggested that Christ's "perfection" through suffering implied some prior lack of holiness. Rather, the hymn contends, Christ's suffering made him "meet" to save sinners. In accordance with Wesley's substitutionary theology of the atonement, the hymn argues that Christ's sufferings are essential for the salvation of the "lost, apostate race." The emphasis on "mine everlasting crown" underlines the personal nature of this sacrifice for the believer.

In the remainder of this hymn, Christ's suffering and death are portrayed as a model for Christian life. Those who follow Christ must also arise "on His cross" and endure "all His pangs." Christ has "consecrated" the way of suffering for believers to follow, so suffering is an appropriate expression of Christian obedience. Those who suffer obediently themselves can confidently expect the benefits of Christ's suffering to apply to them. In the second half of the hymn, these theological contentions are transformed into a prayer: Christ is addressed directly, as the power of "Thy passion" and "Thy blood" is declared. Wesley was careful here to emphasize the primacy of Christ's sufferings in achieving salvation. It is Christ's efforts that provide "peace," "purity" and "pardon" to the believer. Nonetheless, as the last verse contends, these benefits are available only to those who "daily bleed and die with Thee." The "only" way to reach Christ's "glorious throne" is by the "narrow way" of suffering.

The theological argument of this hymn is somewhat convoluted. Wesley carefully sought to establish the significance of Christ's suffering and the necessity of Christian suffering without denying the evangelical axioms of the divinity of Christ and justification by faith. If his argument is complicated, however, its main thrust is straightforward: Christ's suffering is a model for the Christian life. More exactly, the narrative of Christ's suffering, death and resurrection provides a pattern for the Christian life. Christ suffered on the cross – Christians must suffer "on His cross." Christ endured the pangs of death – Christians must endure "all His pangs." After his suffering and death, Christ was resurrected in glory – Christians will, through suffering, be led "to Thy glorious throne." This narrative pattern of suffering followed by glory, derived from the overarching story of Christ's passion and resurrection, dominates Wesley's understanding of the Christian life as explored throughout his hymns. "The cross," as the hymns contend, "shall bring me to the crown."[18]

In presenting Christian life within the narrative structure provided by the story of Christ's suffering and resurrection, Wesley repeatedly employed certain biblical images. Many of these can be seen in a hymn on Mark 10: 38, where Jesus responds to the disciples' request to reign with him in glory.

1. Saviour, who ask to reign with Thee,
They ask (what yet they cannot know)
Thy cup of inward agony,
Thy burden of external woe;
With eagerness of blind desire,
They ask reproach, and pain, and loss,
They ask to be baptized with fire,
And hang expiring on Thy cross.

2. Cover'd with outward sufferings here
Thou wast, with inward sufferings fill'd;
They mark'd Thy perfect character,
They show'd Thee by Thy Father seal'd:
The cross Thou didst for sinners prove

The lot of all Thy followers is;
And leads us on to perfect love,
And paves our way to future bliss.[19]

Here the pattern of Christ's suffering is again presented as normative for Christian life. In both verses of this poem, Wesley made clear his understanding that the follower of Christ must expect to share both the "inward" and "external" or "outward" sufferings of Christ. These sufferings are "The lot of *all* Thy followers."[20] As with Christ, the end result of suffering will be glory: the cross "paves our way to future bliss."

This hymn displays the wide variety of images that Wesley used to explain the meaning of Christ's sufferings and the implications those sufferings have for Christian suffering. The reference to a "cup," following its use in Mark 10: 38, suggests that Christ's sufferings were the cup of God's wrath that Christ drank for sinners.[21] The "burden" that Christ carries may refer to Isaiah 53: 3, which speaks of the Messiah as the one who "hath borne our griefs, and carried our sorrows." Christ's sufferings are described as a baptism of fire, an image also drawn from Mark 10. The hymn implies that believers' sufferings will somehow share these rich and complex meanings. These images of "burden," "cup," "baptism" and "cross," as well as terms related to fire such as "furnace," are all terms that refer to the redemptive purpose of Christ's sufferings. They are shorthand for the whole theology of atonement that informed Wesley's interpretation of the sufferings and death of Christ. He repeatedly used these images to link the sufferings of Christ and the sufferings of Christians. This language provided a rich, metaphorical discourse within which Methodists could describe their sufferings and give them meaning.

Similar images appear in Wesley's poetical commentary on John 1: 37, a verse that reads simply "They followed Jesus."

1. Naked is my heart to Thee:
Would I not Thy follower be?
Tread the path which Thou hast trod,
Track Thee, Saviour, by Thy blood,
Meekly Thine afflictions share,
Every day Thy burden bear,
Drink Thy passion's second cup,
Fill the mournful measure up?

2. Thou didst once for sin atone,
Tread the winepress quite alone,
Yet I may Thy grief partake,
Suffer for my Master's sake,
Through the strength the cross supplies
Mingle with Thy sacrifice,
Bow my head on yonder tree,
Die for One who died for me.[22]

Again, this hymn piles image upon image to communicate Wesley's understanding that the Christian life is one of imitating Jesus in his sufferings all the way to the cross. Some of these images, such as the idea of tracking Jesus by his blood, are vividly original. Others repeat the familiar biblical imagery: while biblical texts might speak of Jesus bearing human burdens, Wesley reversed this image to speak of believers carrying Jesus' burden.[23] The hymn carefully asserts that Christ's sufferings, which "didst *once* for sin atone," are unique. Christians cannot atone for their sins by suffering. Christians may however, "share," "bear," "fill ... up" and "partake" of these sufferings for Christ's sake. The metaphors that describe Christ's sufferings – bearing burdens and drinking bitter cups – can therefore rightly be applied to the suffering of Christians.

These metaphors create a powerful effect of intimacy with Christ, as well as a response of "meekness" or resignation. The hymn repeatedly emphasizes that to suffer as Jesus did is to be close to him: to "track" him, to "drink" his cup, to "mingle" with his sacrifice are images of intense intimacy. The second verse contrasts the pathos of Jesus suffering "quite alone" in his Passion, with the familiarity available to the believer who may now "partake" of Christ's "grief." This intimacy is a result of shared suffering, but it is motivated by the love and gratitude of the narrator, whose heart is "naked" to Christ, and who is willing to "die for One who died for me." The experience of suffering is therefore imbued with powerful emotions of vulnerability, intimacy and love.

In emphasizing the redemptive purposes of Christ's suffering, these images also point to the conviction that Christ suffered deliberately: the language of treading a path, drinking a cup, bearing burdens, treading a winepress suggests active choice, not simply passive acceptance. The narrator of this hymn expresses his or her determination to follow Christ in suffering as he suffered. This is a deliberate choice, which requires "the strength the cross supplies," but it results in "meek" acceptance of resignation in the face of suffering.

As always in Wesley's hymns, the purpose of the hymns considered here is to produce particular emotional and spiritual responses. In the case of these hymns, with their narrative of suffering and reward, the reader or singer is encouraged to internalize this narrative and apply it to his or her own experience. The hymns offered the devout Methodist a vocabulary within which to express and interpret his or her own experiences of suffering. This narrative, and the language through which the believer internalized it, encouraged the believer to understand suffering as an opportunity for imitation of Christ and for intimacy with Christ.

The writings of Methodists certainly suggest an interpretation of personal sufferings within the narrative of Christ's sufferings and a desire to share his attitude of meekness and resignation in the face of suffering. As in the example given at the beginning of this chapter, Sarah Ryan's writings are full of the biblical language found in the hymns. In another letter to her mother she explained:

> As for me I have many trials, but I have scarce time to feel them – my blessed Lord so sweetens every bitter cup. Pray for me that I may lose nothing in the furnace but dross, and stand through all as a beaten anvil to the stroke.[24]

Similarly, writing to Charles in 1740, Ann Martin described her spiritual struggles: "Oh it is a good but painful fight. I was ready to say, 'Father if this cup might pass from me, but thy will be done.'"[25] Susanna Designe wrote to John Wesley on 31 December 1741: "The cup which my Father hath given me, shall I not drink it? Yet can I say, 'Lord, I am in thy hand, do with me what thou wilt, only suffer me not to perish at the last.' Surely there is hope in the end and my expectation shall not be cut off."[26] Margaret Davidson comforted a friend who was being persecuted: "[God] gives you now to partake of the cup of his sorrow but mingles it with love and sweetens it with the joyful prospect of reigning with him for ever."[27] Abraham Jones assured John Wesley: "I want to have the fear of man wholly removed and to be enabled to take up the cross daily and follow Him."[28] In using the imagery of cross and cup to describe their trials, these Methodists gave their physical and emotional pains powerful meanings that identified them with the sufferings of Christ. They appropriated the words of Jesus himself in the face of suffering, and claimed that God was near to them in their experience of pain. They expressed a longing to share Christ's submission in the face of the cross and conveyed a sense of the struggle that it might be not to "shrink" from such suffering.

Wesley's hymns, and the language used by lay Methodists to describe their own lives, support E. P. Thompson's claim that the Methodist "was taught not only to 'bear his Cross' of poverty and humiliation; the crucifixion was... the very pattern of his obedience."[29] As evidence for this claim, Thompson quotes from one of Wesley's hymns: "True followers of our bleeding Lamb, now on Thy daily cross we die." While many of Thompson's conclusions regarding Methodism have been questioned, his analysis here is insightful.[30] He argues that this focus on Christ's suffering had implications for an understanding of life in general, specifically that "Since joy was associated with sin and guilt, and pain (Christ's wounds) with goodness and love, so every impulse became twisted into the reverse." Methodists thus came to believe that people were only approved by God when "performing painful, laborious or self-denying tasks."[31] This twisting of human desires, Thompson contends, in the broader social context of the industrial revolution, meant that Methodist obedience was displayed most immediately in the context of work: "Work was the Cross from which the 'transformed' industrial worker hung."[32]

Thompson is primarily concerned with the second and third generations of Methodists, rather than those of the Wesleys' era. Much of his argument regarding suffering, however, rests on his analysis of Charles Wesley's hymns. Thompson's perceptive observations suggest a number of further questions, the answers to which will shed light on the broader construction of Christian suffering in the hymns. It is clear, as Thompson recognized, that Wesley's hymns encouraged Methodists to see the sufferings of Christ as a model for Christian life. But why? What spiritual purpose did the hymns suggest that this suffering served? What drove the sense of intimacy with Christ and longing for resignation that the hymns communicate? Is Thompson right to take the hymns as representative of Methodist theology and culture? And what were the potential political implications of portraying suffering in these terms?

Sanctification

While the hymns considered above demonstrate Charles Wesley's conviction that Christian suffering should be interpreted with reference to the suffering of Christ, they do not fully explain the understanding behind this conviction. Charles's attitude to suffering in the Christian life is best understood within his broader theology of sanctification, or attainment of personal holiness. The Wesleys' theology of sanctification was one of the most distinctive features of Methodism.[33] This doctrine was also the central issue in a major controversy within the revival in the 1760s, and a point of contention between the Wesley brothers.

As has been suggested by the previous discussion of conversion, Methodist preaching placed a strong emphasis on moral perfection. Both John and Charles Wesley maintained that personal holiness, or "perfection," was the aim of salvation.[34] Prior to their conversions, they understood such perfection as primarily a matter of personal effort. In a sermon composed in 1735, Charles exhorted his hearers: "Christian Perfection is the goal of our religious race; the stand whereon our crown of reward is placed. Hitherto therefore must all our desires be bent; hitherto must all our endeavours tend."[35] Henry Rack suggests that this understanding of the necessity of complete perfection owes much to the Wesleys' early reading of Jeremy Taylor, Thomas a Kempis and William Law.[36] These writers emphasized the importance of an "inward" holiness that went beyond right actions to involve the subjection of the entire self to God.[37] This notion of "inward holiness" was the standard against which the Wesleys would continue to judge the human heart.

In the context of the theological shifts that accompanied their conversions, the brothers came to see the place of moral perfection differently. They accepted the idea of "imputed righteousness," in which the justified sinner was not only forgiven for sin, but was credited by God with the righteousness of Christ. Charles expressed this idea in his famous work "And Can it Be?" in the words: "No condemnation now I dread;/ Jesus, and all in him, is mine!/ Alive in him, my living head,/ And clothed in righteousness divine."[38] While justification, including the imputation of Christ's righteousness, meant that believers were no longer required to earn salvation through personal effort, the Wesleys continued to teach that holiness was the ultimate aim of salvation. In a sermon preached after his conversion, Charles contended, "Holiness is the test and evidence, no less than the end of faith… If Christ is made unto me righteousness, he is, he must be, made unto me sanctification also. His righteousness is not imputed to me, unless I manifest it by righteousness also."[39]

This understanding of sanctification reflected the doctrine of "recapitulation," which has been discussed in the previous chapter. According to this doctrine, the purpose of salvation was the re-formation of the image of God, understood as moral perfection, in humanity. Being "born again" was the beginning of the process by which God's image was restored in an individual. The "end" of this process was the transformation of the character of the individual to become like God or, more specifically, Christ.[40] Crucially, however, the experience of conversion taught Methodists that they were powerless to resist sin through their own strength. This ability was given by God in conversion, but only to those who continued to depend on him, hence Wesley's assurance that holiness was the "test and evidence" of faith. Only those in whose hearts Christ "lived and reigned" could be exhorted to strive for holiness.[41]

Both John and Charles agreed, therefore, that true justification should and must result in sanctification. They agreed that at conversion the individual was given a new power to resist sin. But their ideas on how, and to what degree, this sanctification was achieved in the Christian life brought them into conflict with each other, and with others within the evangelical movement.[42] Controversially, the Wesley brothers taught that "entire sanctification" was possible in this life. Their views on exactly what such sanctification involved seem to have shifted over time, influenced by their own experience, the experience of Methodists who claimed to have gained perfection and the ongoing theological debates within evangelical circles more broadly.[43] By the 1760s, John was teaching that believers could receive an instantaneous gift of entire sanctification, much as they had received the gift of justification. This gift allowed them to love God and their neighbor perfectly, though they would not, in this life, be free from temptation or "infirmities." John argued that many Methodists could testify to this experience, and he collected and scrutinized accounts of their experience.[44] Sarah Ryan was a leading example of a Methodist who claimed entire sanctification during this period.

While Charles shared John's belief in the possibility of entire sanctification, he seems to have maintained an unqualified view of this gift: those who received it would be free from *all* temptation and fault. He concluded that very few Christians achieved this state and that it was only given, through a lengthy process of spiritual maturing, to those on the point of death.[45] This stricter definition of perfection may have resulted in part from a reaction to the "perfectionist" revivals of the 1760s, when hundreds of Methodists claimed to have received entire sanctification. Charles was suspicious of these claims, and the revivals eventually resulted in the secession of a number of Methodists from the Wesleys. In hymns written around this time Charles poured scorn on the idea that perfection could be so easily achieved:

> Go on? But how? From step to step?
> No: let us to perfection leap!
> 'Tis thus our hasty nature cries,
> Leap o'er the cross, to snatch the prize,
> Like *Jonah's* gourd, displays its bower,
> And blooms, and withers in an hour.[46]

More sympathetic to the claimants to perfection, John criticized his brother for this view:

> One word more, concerning setting perfection too high. That perfection which I believe, I can boldly preach, because I think I see five hundred witnesses of it. Of that perfection which you preach, you do not even see any witnesses at all.

> Why, then you must have far more courage than me, or you could not persist in preaching it.[47]

In spite of this criticism, Charles wrote hymns promoting a "high" view of perfection throughout his life.[48]

The differences between the brothers' views will be considered in more detail shortly. Their shared convictions about the importance and possibility of holiness had, however, a significant impact on the Methodist understanding of the Christian life. In particular, Rack contends, they created "an extended scenario for the drama of salvation which became distinctive of Wesleyanism, offering the believer a pilgrim's progress from sin through conviction, through conversion, to perfection and beyond."[49] The typical Methodist conversion narrative described an "awakening" and a painful struggle against sin, followed by the transformative experience of conversion. The hymns point, however, to a broader narrative culture within Methodism, in which individual believers understood all the events of their lives as forming a story of enormous spiritual significance. The Wesleys' understanding of sanctification meant that for them the initial transformation of conversion was followed by a life of continued struggle toward the higher goal of entire sanctification.

This narrative encouraged Methodists to believe both that they had been decisively delivered from sin and that they must still struggle against it. It encouraged Methodists to perceive that they were both helpless to save themselves and empowered to work toward perfection. It encouraged Methodists to see the transformation of their souls as a result of both their own daily choices and a sovereign work of God to which they must submit. Phyllis Mack has argued that this deep tension within Methodism was partially countered by the emphasis in Methodist hymns on the suffering of Christ. Wesley's depictions of the bleeding and vulnerable Jesus were a powerful reminder of believers' dependence on his love and sacrifice.[50] More broadly, this tension between dependence and agency is resolved in Wesley's hymns through a construction of sanctification that gives a central place to suffering.

Suffering and Submission

Wesley contended that the character of Christ was formed in an individual as he or she "denied self" and submitted to the will of God. For Wesley, the suffering of Christ was the perfect expression of such self-denial and submission. By following in his footsteps, Christians could also achieve these attitudes. This understanding was clearly expressed in a hymn based on Hebrews 12: 10.

> 1. Father, that we are truly Thine,
> By Thine afflicting hand we know,
> Enter into Thy kind design,
> Partakers with the Man of woe,
> And bear our lot of sacred pain,
> Thy nature, and Thy throne to' obtain.

2. Though slow of heart, we comprehend
The gracious meaning of Thy rod,
Who dost in every stroke intend
Our spiritual, eternal good:
We bless Thine acceptable will,
Which scourges and afflicts us still.

3. The good, which we could never find
Untroubled, unchastised by Thee,
We feel, in pain and grief resign'd,
The patient, meek humility,
The mind, which in our Saviour was,
And all the bearers of His cross

4. Then let us still His cross sustain,
A Father's chastisements receive,
And waiting thus the prize to gain,
We shall the life Divine retrieve,
And put Thy sinless image on,
Pure members of Thy perfect Son.[51]

Here the purpose of suffering is to create in the believer "the mind, which in our Saviour was." This "mind" is one of resignation and "patient, meek humility." In the face of terrible suffering, Christ was able to submit to his Father with the words, "Not my will, but Thine be done." Through suffering his followers can also demonstrate and develop this submission to "Thine acceptable will." The "good" of this submissive heart could not be achieved other than through the experience of "pain and grief." As the last verse makes explicit, it is through this process of humbly submitting to the "Father's chastisements" that the "sinless image" of God is re-formed in the individual. This is "the crown" to which "the cross" leads.

Suffering, then, is the means by which the self is brought into complete submission. As the previous hymn suggests, Wesley identified such suffering as "chastisement." Even in the life of the believer, suffering retained its primary meaning of judgment against sin. For the believer, however, God's chastisements were given in love and are effective in bringing about change. This can be seen in a hymn for one "In Temptation."

1. Glory to the righteous God,
Righteous, yet benign to me!
Still in His paternal rod
His paternal love I see:
Let Him tenderly chastise,
Let Him graciously reprove,
Father, all within me cries
All Thy ways are truth and love.

2. Humbled in the lowest deep,
Thee I for my sufferings bless;
Think of all Thy love, and weep
For my own unfaithfulness:
I have most rebellious been,
Thou hast laid Thine hand on me,
Kindly visited my sin,
Scourged the wanderer back to Thee.

3. Taught obedience to my God,
By the things I have endured,
Meekly now I kiss the rod,
Wounded by the rod, and cured:
Good for me the grief and pain,
Let me but Thy grace adore,
Keep the pardon I regain,
Stand in awe, and sin no more.[52]

Here, suffering is God's disciplinary "rod" but it is also a sign of his fatherly "love." God's punishment is inflicted "tenderly," "graciously" and with "kindly" intent. The narrator testifies that this suffering "wounded" the self and in doing so "cured" it. The self is constructed as rebellious and unfaithful, and desperately in need of correction. Suffering is the instrument that can provide this cure. As this hymn makes explicit, it is the ability of suffering to chasten and transform the "inner world" of the heart that makes it so powerful as an instrument of sanctification. Here the believer is taught humility, repentance, meekness and awe by "the rod" of suffering. By maintaining these attitudes, the believer may "keep the pardon I regain" and so "sin no more."

Wesley's hymns, therefore, present the Christian life as an ongoing battle between the sinful self and the goal of submission. This ultimate goal is achievable only by means of suffering. A detailed description of this process is given in one of his early hymns, entitled "A Welcome to the Cross" (see Hymn 3). This hymn begins with a welcome to the "hallowed cross," which is clearly an ongoing experience of suffering. Whether this is an external affliction, or simply the experience of self-denial, is not clear. This counterintuitive attitude to suffering is reinforced by a detailed narrative that describes the battle for sanctification within the believer: a battle in which suffering is the only effective weapon. From the beginning of the poem, sanctification is portrayed as requiring significant violence: Christ is called upon to "wither," "destroy," "stain," "implunge," "kill," "cut off," "pluck out" and "tear" aspects of the sinful self.

Verses three to six describe the inner state of the narrator – rebelling against Christ and repressing the soul. Each verse follows the same pattern: a lament over the stubbornness of the sinful self, followed by a call for Christ to apply the weapon of suffering to bring about the destruction of this self. The repetition of this pattern suggests an ongoing battle, in which repeated attempts to destroy "the self" are followed by repeated recognition that "the self" still survives. The narrator longs for Christ, rather than self, to be in control. This can only be brought about, as the first and last verses make clear, if the person suffers until the sinful self is put to death. Only then will the individual be resurrected, like Christ, "Partaker of a life Divine."

This hymn has much in common with Wesley's hymns on the experience of struggling against sin before conversion. The inner self of the individual is depicted as deeply conflicted; the "will," "pride" and "nature's life" of the individual still rebel against God; the "soul" still struggles and the "heart" still requires breaking. Yet the situation in this hymn is noticeably different from that depicted in the hymns for those mourning before conversion. The narrator in these hymns has a confident assurance that Christ will act in his or her life. This action is, primarily, the application of "the cross" of suffering to bring about the death of the sinful will. Through this "cross" the sinful self will be crucified and the power of Christ will more fully control the believer. Where before conversion the individual mourned over the painful experience of sin, here the experience of pain is welcomed as a sign of the presence and power of Christ.

Sanctification, therefore, was not simply a negative experience, by which the selfish nature was put to death, but also a positive experience, by which this nature was replaced by the loving character of Christ. For Wesley, as for many other Methodists, achieving this transformed nature was worth any price:

> This, this is the one thing needful – not a friend, not health, not life itself – but the pure, perfect love of Christ Jesus. O give me love, or else I die! O give me love, and let me die! I am weary of my want of love – weary to death, and would fain throw off this body, that I may love him who so loved me.[53]

It is in the context of this desire for a transformed nature that Wesley's emphasis on the value of suffering must be seen. Suffering was the means by which the character of Christ was formed. A hymn "For a Sick Friend" urges Christ to "Enter his heart, possess him whole./ Inspire and actuate his soul;/ Himself no longer let it be/ That suffers, or that lives – but Thee."[54] Suffering provided the circumstance in which Christ could take possession of the self.

Wesley thus distinguished between suffering as an instrument of sanctification, and Christ as the one who wields this instrument.

> Can sufferings purge my inbred sin?
> No more than it can heaven procure:
> But He, who brought this fire within,
> By patience makes my nature pure.
> But He, who with the suffering comes,
> My dross in His own way consumes.
>
> His love into the furnace cast.
> His love attends and keeps me here,
> That coming forth as gold at last,
> Stamp'd with His name and character,
> And perfected through sufferings I
> May spotless to His bosom fly.[55]

Suffering alone is not effective, these verses suggest, but "He, who with the suffering comes" makes use of the suffering for spiritual benefit. The second verse suggests an image of Christ as goldsmith – casting the believer into the furnace, keeping the believer there until he or she is purified "as gold," stamping the believer with "His name and character." Christ brings the suffering, accompanies it with his presence and his love, forms his own character in the sufferer through it and welcomes the sufferer at its ceasing.

For Wesley, then, the experience of lifelong suffering was the means by which the Christian was able to progress toward sanctification without becoming sinfully reliant on self. The experience of suffering repeatedly reminded the believer of his or her weakness and dependence. In the "furnace" of physical, spiritual or emotional pain, the believer would rely on the power of Christ, who would enable the believer to submit with resignation to God's will. The agency of the believer was exercised through the repeated decision to submit to Christ. The presence of Christ and the memory of his suffering would make this experience one of loving intimacy with him.

The conviction that suffering was part of God's good work in the believer explains how Wesley's emphasis on suffering could be accompanied, throughout the hymns, by an emphasis on joy. As Wesley wrote in a typical hymn "for Believers":

> 3. Jesu, my all in all thou art,
> My rest in toil, my ease in pain;
> The med'cine of my broken heart,
> In war my peace, in loss my gain;
> My smile beneath the tyrant's frown,
> In shame my glory and my crown.
>
> 4. In want my plentiful supply,
> In weakness my almighty power;
> In bonds my perfect liberty,
> My light in Satan's darkest hour;
> In grief my joy unspeakable,
> My life in death, my heaven in hell.[56]

For the believer, the suffering of pain, loss, shame, grief and death could all be accompanied by "joy unspeakable" because such hardships did not detract from – but rather added to – the assurance of the presence of Christ and the love of God.

Early Methodist writings demonstrate that many men and women welcomed affliction for its spiritual benefits. Elizabeth Sais testified in May 1742: "I have gone through close trials which always worked together for my good, for I found that temptation always stirred me up to lay hold on the Lord, for suffering faith did always brighter glow and purify the heart."[57] Susanna Designe wrote to John Wesley in a time of suffering: "If I could believe I was in the fiery furnace, my sufferings would be nothing for then I know my Lord would bring me forth as gold tried in the fire."[58] Longing for sanctification, Mary Maddern prophesied that "there was a larger measure of sufferings for me before I am made an inhabitant of that [good land]; though it is what I both look for and long for."[59]

bitant of that [good land]; though it is what I both look for and long for."[59] These women shared the perspective of the hymns in asserting that suffering could be welcomed as a blessing, if it was part of God's purifying work in the believer. This understanding did not lead the women to a masochistic delight in pain, but to an acceptance of suffering as the necessary means by which God would bring about their sanctification.

As Susanna Designe's words imply, however, suffering did not automatically result in purification. For those who rejected God's grace, suffering retained its primary and permanent meaning of judgment.[60] Wesley's few hymns on hell make clear his understanding that it was a place where "all the power of hellish pains" would torment the unrepentant sinner forever.[61] But Designe's letter demonstrates that even the devout believer could fear that their pain might be "unhallow'd."

Wesley's hymns encouraged Methodist women and men to expect and welcome affliction as the path to sanctification. This theme is repeated throughout his hymns, though it appears more often and more explicitly in the hymns written after the perfection controversies of the 1760s.[62] Wesley's increasing emphasis on suffering may have reflected these controversies, or perhaps his own ongoing experience of depression, illness, bereavement and disappointment. Whatever the reason, his hymns presented the pattern of Christ's suffering, rewarded by resurrection and glory, as a narrative structure on which Christians could plot their road to perfection. Those who read and sang Wesley's hymns were encouraged to internalize this narrative and adopt a biblically derived language of cup, cross, burden and fire to describe their own experiences. The hymns assured believers that in the midst of suffering they could experience intimacy with Christ and spiritual growth – and the writings of Methodist laypeople confirm that they often understood their experience in these terms. But to what extent did the more unusual aspects of Wesley's construction of suffering reflect a broader Methodist understanding?

Conflicting Views

Charles Wesley's conviction that suffering was a valuable and even necessary part of Christian discipleship was not historically unusual. Orthodox Christian theology had always taught that suffering was the result of human sinfulness, but God, in his love, would still use it for the good of those who served him.[63] Theologians had explained the value of suffering in different ways. The medieval church taught that because of Christ's suffering, as well as the suffering of the martyrs and the suffering of ordinary Christians who sacrificed themselves in daily obedience, the church was able to intercede with God for individual human beings. From the store of merit accumulated through this suffering, the church was able to grant indulgences to repentant believers, delivering them from the future suffering of purgatory.[64]

The Reformers, by contrast, denied any salvational worth to human actions, as well as the mediating role of the church.[65] Human hope for salvation must instead be placed fully in the meritorious suffering of the "crucified God," as Martin Luther described Christ. Reformation theology, both in its Lutheran and Calvinist formulations, emphasized the sovereignty of God in all things. Human suffering was part of God's providence, and should be accepted as part of his good, if mysterious purposes. There was spiritual benefit in suffering, both Luther and Calvin suggested, because it taught virtues such as patience, and encouraged the believer to have faith in God alone.[66]

As a theological heir of the Reformers, Wesley was careful to emphasize that it was Christ's sufferings and death alone that brought salvation. In his general emphasis on God's sovereignty in human suffering and the resulting spiritual benefit of such suffering, Wesley also followed standard Reformation theology. The emphasis within the hymns on the imitative quality of Christian suffering was also not unusual. Biblical passages that taught the value of suffering provided a common basis for such theologies.[67]

As has been suggested, however, the Wesleys' theology of perfection was innovative, and Charles's insistence on the necessity of extreme suffering as the means to perfection is distinctive. This can be seen in the way the hymns considered here make use of Christ's command to his disciples in Mark 8: 34, "Whosoever will come after me, let him deny himself, and take up his cross, and follow me." Wesley often followed this passage in describing Christian life and discipleship in terms of the cross. Significantly, however, where the biblical passage refers to each follower taking up "his" own cross, Wesley repeatedly referred to followers bearing *Christ's* cross. So, in the examples above, the believer expects to "hang expiring on *Thy* cross," welcomes "*the Saviour's* hallow'd cross" and longs to share "the sufferings of *Thy* cross." Whereas in the biblical passage "taking up his cross" could be understood as a matter of self-denial, in Wesley's interpretation it became a matter of suffering as Christ suffered. As E. P. Thompson perceptively recognized, Wesley went beyond a conventional Christian emphasis on "bearing the cross" of particular hardships, to suggesting that the cross provided the pattern, or narrative, of the Christian life. It is this interpretation, and its implications in the poems, that causes Tyson to contend that "Charles Wesley extended the atonement into the daily life of Christians as few Protestant theologians have dared."[68]

Wesley's insistence on the need for Christians to suffer as Christ suffered can be seen in his portrayal of the "wilderness state." Following an idea common among medieval mystics such as St. John of the Cross, Wesley contended that God would sometimes withdraw his presence from believers so as to test and strengthen their faith.[69] One of many hymns Wesley wrote on this theme was an unpublished hymn on Mark 2: 19–20.

3. No abstinence severe
Can be, while Christ is here:
High on eagles' wings we soar,
Safe in heavenly places dwell;
War and strife we reckon o'er,
Suffering is impossible.

4. But soon or late we moan
Our joyous Bridegroom gone,
Miss that sensible delight,
Extasy of infant grace,
Lose the Beatific Sight,
See no more his heavenly face.

5. His face unless he hide,
We never can be tried:
Wherefore not in wrath but love
Jesus partially withdraws,
Leaves his own, our faith to prove,
Leaves us bleeding on his cross.[70]

In this narrative, the Christian experience is one of initial joy after conversion, followed inevitably by spiritual suffering as the presence of Christ is "partially" withdrawn. Particularly in his later hymns, Wesley repeatedly suggested that this experience was normative.[71] Wesley's emphasis on this experience of abandonment complicates his portrayal of suffering as an experience of intimacy with Christ, by introducing the possibility of a new category of suffering: the suffering of absence. The language of this hymn suggests, however, that in this experience the believer imitates Christ, who cried out on the cross that God had abandoned him. Wesley wrote multiple hymns in which he encouraged Methodists to believe that, in order to imitate Christ fully, they must endure such an experience of abandonment.[72]

The distinctiveness of Charles's interpretation is demonstrated by examining John's somewhat different understanding. In a sermon "On Self-Denial," John dealt explicitly with the question of "taking up the cross" to follow Jesus:

> A cross is anything contrary to our will, anything displeasing to our nature... We are then properly said to "bear our cross" when we endure what is laid upon us without our choice, with meekness and resignation. Whereas, we do not properly "take up our cross", but when we voluntarily suffer what it is in our power to avoid; when we willingly embrace the will of God, though contrary to our own.[73]

This description affirms many aspects of Charles's understanding of the place of suffering in the Christian life. To "endure what is laid upon us without our choice, with meekness and resignation" and "to voluntarily suffer what it is in our power to avoid" are both given great spiritual significance. Notably, however, John outlined a narrative of the Christian life that differs from that provided by Charles's hymns:

> Now, in running "the race which is set before us," according to the will of God, there is often a cross lying in the way; that is, something which is not only not joyous, but grievous; something which is contrary to our will... What then is to be done? The choice is plain: Either we must take up our cross, or we must turn away from the way of God.[74]

For John, the pattern of life was a race, in which "our cross" must often be taken up in order to faithfully follow the will of God. He did not conclude, however, that the cross of Christ was the pattern for the whole of life, or that Christians must suffer to the extent that Christ suffered.

John's thoughts on the place of suffering in the Christian life can also be seen in two sermons entitled "The Wilderness State" and "Heaviness through Manifold Temptations," written in 1760. John's primary focus in these sermons was the spiritual meanings of religious anxiety and depression. In discussing this issue, however, John also dealt more generally with the meaning and purpose of suffering for the Christian. Like his brother, he saw great potential spiritual value in suffering, particularly because it contributed to "holiness" or complete submission to God: "sanctified afflictions have (through the grace of God) an immediate and direct tendency to holiness. Through the operation of his Spirit they humble more and more, and abase the soul before God."[75] John argued, however, that the biblical reference to trials through which believers may share the "sufferings of Christ" did not refer to general sufferings. From the context of the passage he argued that this phrase "doubtless refers to martyrdom and the sufferings connected with it."[76]

Further, John was careful to affirm that constant suffering was not a necessity for the Christian. Commenting on 1 Peter 1: 6, which reads, "Now for a season, if need be, ye are in heaviness through manifold temptations," John wrote:

> From the Apostle's manner of speaking we may gather, thirdly, that even heaviness is not *always* needful... it is not needful for *all persons*; nor for any person at *all times*. God is able... to work when he pleases the same work of grace, in any soul, by other means. And in some instances he does so: he causes those whom it pleaseth him to go on from strength to strength... But these cases are rare... manifold temptations and heaviness, more or less, are usually the portion of his dearest children.[77]

For John, then, suffering was beneficial and common, but not necessary or constant. And there was no place for considering all the daily hardships of the Christian's life as the sufferings of Christ.

In his sermon on "The Wilderness State," John directly contradicted Charles's understanding of that experience. While John agreed that Christians could *feel* deserted by God, he contended that God "never deserts us, as some speak: it is we only that desert him."[78] If a believer felt deserted by God, John argued, it must be the result of unrepented sin or of some physical or emotional malady. In a possible reference to his brother, John continued:

> If men... imagine there are passages either in the Old or New Testament which assert that all believers without exception must sometimes be in darkness, this ignorance will naturally bring upon them the darkness which they expect. And how common a case has this been among us!... Not only the mystic writers of the Romish Church, but many of the most spiritual and experimental in our own... lay it down with all assurance.[79]

Rather, John contended: "Joy in the Holy Ghost will far more effectually purify the soul than the want of that joy."[80]

The theological differences between the brothers on these points are most obvious in John's comments on Charles's poems. John marked his copy of Charles's *Short Hymns on Select Passages of Scripture* with a number of queries and exclamations, and most of these comments relate to the question of suffering in the believer's life. A typical example is Charles's hymn on Hebrews 12: 8, a verse that reads, "But if ye be without chastisement, whereof all are partakers, then are ye bastards, and not sons."

1. The children every one partake
The chastisement for all design'd,
Their God doth no exception make
Impartially, severely kind,
No favourite uncorrected leaves,
But scourges all whom He receives.

2. To none of the believing race
This mark their Father's love denies:
But when he sees the light of grace
The babe in Christ that moment cries,*
And of the heavenly Spirit born
Begins at once to breathe, and mourn.

3. In sorrow, as in grace, we grow,
With closer fellowship in pain,
Our Lord more intimately know,
Till coming to a perfect man
His sharpest agonies we share,*
And all His marks of passion bear.

4. Partakers of His bitterest cup,
And burden'd with His heaviest load,
We fill His after-sufferings up,
Conform'd to an expiring God;
And only such our Father owns,*
And seats on our appointed thrones.[81]

This poem repeats the narrative pattern in which the story of the Christian's life is one of increasing suffering culminating in glorious reward. Christian maturity in this life is connected to experiencing the extremes of Christ's suffering. The asterisks indicate points at which John inserted the comment "No!" in his copy of the poems. George Osborn, the nineteenth-century editor of *The Poetical Works of John and Charles Wesley*, remarks on these insertions: "Wesley's repeated 'No,' will be echoed by every judicious reader in regard not only to the time and degree, but also to the universal necessity of such suffering as is here, and in several other places, spoken of."[82]

Charles's assertions that suffering was the first experience of "the babe in Christ"; that the Christian shared Christ's "sharpest agonies"; and that "only such" Christians as partook of these sufferings would be accepted by God, were firmly opposed by his brother, as well as by Methodists such as Osborn. As has already been mentioned, John criticized his brother for the "gloomy cast" of his mind and verse and for frequently describing religion as "a melancholy thing."[83] The divergence between John and Charles on these points represented not only a different theology of sanctification, but alternative normative narratives of the Christian experience. For John, the Christian life was not "a melancholy thing": severe trials were to be expected, but cheerfulness was the norm and the delights of perfection were a real possibility.[84] Life was a demanding race, not a slow crucifixion. For Charles, however, the Christian should not expect perfection before the moment of death. In the meantime, life was a matter of intense and increasing suffering, involving physical and emotional pains as well as the spiritual pain of being abandoned by God. Joy was certainly a reality, but it was experienced as a loving intimacy with Christ in the midst of pain and as a confident hope of eternity ahead.

While the difference between the brothers was for the most part one of degrees, rather than absolute disagreement, recognizing this distinction complicates the picture of Methodism painted by E. P. Thompson. In particular, it disturbs his portrayal of a movement in which a unified, strictly controlled, "orthodox" body of doctrine and practice represented the real Methodism, and alternative expressions within Methodism are aberrations reflecting "plain common-sense, compassion, [and] the obstinate vitality of older community traditions."[85] The Wesleys' differences demonstrate that early Methodist culture contained (at least) two "orthodox" constructions of the relationship between suffering and Christian obedience. That the nineteenth-century Methodist editor of Charles Wesley's works felt it necessary to express his disapproval of Charles's emphasis on suffering suggests that Charles's construction was frowned upon during this period – but the offending hymns were still published.[86]

As Hempton and Walsh have argued, however, any analysis of Methodist culture must go beyond a "top-down" approach.[87] Methodist attitudes to suffering cannot simply be read from the sermons of John or the hymns of Charles. Without attempting an extensive analysis of these broader attitudes, early Methodist writings provide evidence of a more complicated engagement with the various "orthodoxies" than Thompson's depiction would suggest.

The writings and autobiographical account of Sarah Ryan are a particularly rich source of such evidence. On one occasion, Mary Bosanquet recorded, Ryan was challenged by another Methodist, who believed that Ryan's intense spiritual struggles showed she was not truly sanctified.

> [Ryan] answered little but carried it to the Lord – when it was shown her the Holy Lamb of God *suffered* being tempted, and that the apostle makes that remark for our comfort. And that it was said by our Lord "he shall indeed drink of my cup and be baptised with my baptism." And considering Mr Wesley's note on those words, "the cup of his *inward* and the baptism of his *outward* sufferings", her soul was greatly refreshed and comforted.[88]

Bosanquet's account provides a compelling example of the way in which understandings about suffering were debated within early Methodism. The unnamed woman who challenged Ryan believed that sanctification would relieve the believer of spiritual struggle. Ryan's opposing understanding, which she believed was "shown her" by God, drew upon both Scriptural texts and a quote from John Wesley's *Explanatory Notes* on Scripture.

Ryan also used Charles's hymns in developing her understanding of suffering. Many of the passages on suffering in her writings contain quotes from Charles Wesley's hymns. She often used a phrase of Wesley's that equated suffering and obedience: "Jesus I come thy will to do/ I come thy will to suffer, too."[89] She urged her sister Phebe, "nothing would be a greater grief to me than to have your troubles drive you from God. Pray much and they never shall, but like Moses's bush you will mount the higher and flourish unconsumed in fire." The latter phrase comes from *Hymns and Sacred Poems* (1739).

These passages show that Ryan drew on a number of sources in constructing her response to suffering, among them Scripture, John Wesley's writings and the hymns of Charles Wesley. However her own understanding of suffering was not simply a carbon copy of either brother's interpretation. Her claim to have received full sanctification put her at odds with Charles Wesley's belief that such perfection was received only at the end of life. The centrality of suffering to her spiritual experience and her almost ecstatic welcome of such pain was, however, more in keeping with Charles's model of Christian life than with John's. Like Charles, she was convinced that she would suffer continuously until the end of her life, a conviction that arose from a vision that she believed God had given her.[90] For Ryan, this personal revelation and her own interpretation of Scripture were as authoritative as the opinions of the Wesley brothers. The resulting narrative she constructed for her life drew on both brothers' teaching, but was not a carbon copy of either.

A similar diversity of views within early Methodism can be seen in attitudes to the "wilderness experience" among Methodists. Many Methodists who wrote to Charles described experiences of emotional and spiritual trial, which they often described as "darkness that can be felt."[91] Like Charles, they interpreted these experiences as the withdrawal of God's presence, in ways that would have been unacceptable to John. For these believers, the idea of the "wilderness experience" made sense of their experience in a way that John's more matter-of-fact explanation did not.

Methodist laypeople did not always affirm with Charles that a continual, intense experience of suffering was necessary for sanctification. However, their different responses to suffering encourage a view of Methodist culture that recognizes that believers were not simply brainwashed by a unified elite, but were agents who chose between different perspectives offered by the Methodist leadership and others.[92]

While Charles's more extreme ideas about suffering may not have become part of mainstream Methodist conviction (and certainly, most of his hymns on suffering were only rarely reproduced after his death) the narrative of Christian life that he emphasized was an enduring one. A. Gregory Schneider argues that "the way of the cross" was a central metaphor for understanding life in early American Methodist culture. He disagrees, however, with E. P. Thompson's claims, noting that "The important rhetorical feature of the way of the cross... was not the *association* of pain with pleasure but the *sequence* or *progression* from pain and suffering to pleasure and joy."[93] That is, devout Methodists took courage from the belief that temporary suffering would, by God's grace, be transformed into eternal joy. Schneider concludes that Thompson's "associationist psychology" prevents him from recognizing this "diachronic, narrative element in Methodist piety."[94] While Schneider does not explore Wesley's hymns as a source of this narrative element, his criticism of Thompson's analysis is insightful. Both John and Charles Wesley taught that suffering would lead to joy, but it was Charles's hymns that placed this theological conviction in narratives that were repeatedly read and sung by Methodist believers.

Bearing the Cross and Bearing Injustice

E. P. Thompson's argument is more closely concerned, however, with the passive acceptance of injustice that he believes the hymns perpetuated. If all of life's sufferings could be seen as "a cross," and thus a burden to be accepted with resignation, did the hymns implicitly encourage Methodists to respond passively to the social and economic status quo? Early Methodist writings suggest that the attitudes toward suffering contained in the hymns certainly could encourage a meek acceptance of injustice. Again, one possible example of the attitude to suffering modeled in the hymns is found in the writings of Sarah Ryan. Following her conversion, Ryan began to interpret her husband's violence toward her as God's righteous punishment for her previous sins:

> Mr. Ryan came home again, and my sufferings were great, but resistance was over. The iron sinew in my neck was broke, and I read my sin in every punishment, and adored God for his justice as well as his mercy, quietly taking the most barbarous treatment![95]

Understanding the violence of her husband as a punishment from God (though still recognizing it as "barbarous treatment"), Ryan chose not to resist it. In the context, her lack of resistance is portrayed as a Christ-like response of resignation. Certainly, then, combined with a politically conservative theology, the attitudes to suffering modeled in Wesley's hymns could lead to introspection and political quietism.

It is inadequate, however, to suggest that the hymns simply encouraged a passive acceptance of suffering. Rather, as has been argued, by modeling the believer's response to suffering upon Christ's, they portrayed this response to suffering as an active one. If suffering was a tool of God in the believer's life, it was the believer's responsibility to respond rightly to the painful experience, ascertaining its spiritual meaning and struggling to develop the correct attitude toward it. This was, ultimately, a question of submitting to God. It was not necessarily submission to injustice. Sarah Ryan, who so meekly accepted her husband's beatings, later decided that God was calling her to leave the marriage, against her desire to remain.[96] She went on to become an influential Methodist leader and preacher.

The narrative contained in Wesley's hymns – of radical transformation into a life of submission to God – was, as E. P. Thompson recognized, inherently political. It involved a change in the individual's perceptions of, and response to, authority. It did not, however, necessarily lead to a passive acceptance of injustice. This can particularly be seen in the experience of the second and third generations of Methodist women, some of whom were members of the generation of Methodists that Thompson saw as having deeply internalized a theology of political and personal submission. The writings of these women suggest otherwise. For example, at the annual Methodist Conference in 1809, the assembled preachers revisited a long-standing debate over the propriety of women preachers. In spite of vehement opposition from some of those present, the Conference agreed not to restrict women's preaching further.[97] Mary Taft, the most famous Methodist woman preacher of her time and focus of much of the controversy, observed the debate. At its conclusion, she rejoiced:

> This was a time of trial to me, but our God overruled. Praise his holy name for ever! I felt and prayed much for myself, family, friends, and the church of God. The Lord preserve me from shrinking from the Cross, but may we glory in it and live under it till we change it for a crown.[98]

Taft interpreted her experience of opposition to women's ministry within the narrative of "cross" and "crown." This motivated her, however, to continue to persevere in her preaching, against much opposition. For Taft, to "glory under" the cross was not to accept injustice, but to embrace suffering as the necessary cost of faithful discipleship. Faithful discipleship could include the confronting of perceived injustice or the transgressing of social norms. John Wesley himself had encouraged such an understanding, writing to Mary Bishop, a Methodist woman anxious about speaking in public: "Take up your cross; when the occasion offers, break through, speak, though it is pain and grief unto you."[99]

The same attitude can be found in the writings of Dorothy Ripley, a Methodist woman who traveled alone from Whitby to America in 1801 to campaign against slavery. Ripley spent the next thirty years working against slavery, crossing the Atlantic multiple times, addressing Congress and confronting slaveholders, starting schools for ex-slaves and eventually campaigning on behalf of prisoners and Native Americans.[100] Starting out on her first journey to America, she wrote in a prayer, "And if great suffering be my allotment to ally me to thee, never let me shrink from the bitter cup offered in mercy."[101] For Ripley, the conviction that "great suffering" was a means of achieving greater intimacy with Christ helped provide ongoing motivation for withstanding the pains and demands of a life of activism.

These examples suggest that this construction of the Christian life could be especially meaningful for Methodist women who, as Mack argues, were particularly exposed to suffering through childbirth and their role as primary carers of the sick and bereaved.[102] The road to sanctification that the hymns depict, in which submission and suffering are central, was accessible to these women through their daily experience, even if they did not share Sarah Ryan's experience of terrible domestic violence. This had the potential both to give women such as Ryan a new spiritual authority as exemplars of the ideal and to motivate women such as Mary Taft and Dorothy Ripley to activism that challenged conventional gender boundaries. The history of eighteenth- and nineteenth-century Methodism suggests that both of these occurred, in ways that at times expanded, and at times limited, the opportunities for women in the movement.[103]

Wesley's hymns encouraged Methodist believers to expect a life of suffering that paralleled the sufferings of Christ. Such suffering would be agonizing and overwhelming but, by the power of Christ, would result in the purification and perfection of the self. The cross of suffering would result in the crown of eternal reward. As this chapter has demonstrated, aspects of this portrayal of suffering were controversial within Methodism, and early Methodists clearly did not adopt Wesley's construction wholesale. The basic construction of suffering contained in the hymns, however, helps explain one of the tensions at the heart of the movement, which combined a broad political conservatism with significant missionary and reformist activism. Wesley's hymns provided Methodists with an interpretative framework that could require a resigned acceptance of injustice, but could also sustain a life of activism against injustice. The next chapter explores how the hymns also acted as tools to assist Methodists in the difficult task of responding to individual experiences of suffering.

[Hymn 1]
Groaning for Redemption (Part I)

1. Lord, I confess my sins to Thee,
My sins beyond expression great;
Fast bound in sin and misery,
My spirit faints beneath the weight,
And struggles to throw off the load,
But cannot, cannot come to God.

2. O how shall I the anguish bear
Of inbred sin's invenomed dart?
The mischief hence I cannot tear,
'Tis enter'd deep within my heart,
Its poison drinks my spirits up,
And quenches my last spark of hope.

3. O wretched man, what must I do?
I neither can resist nor fly;
Hell, earth, and sin my soul pursue,
I cannot find my Saviour nigh;
Unhappy, I shall one day fall,
Shall perish by the hand of *Saul*.

4. Me from perdition what can save?
Justly my God His help denies:
No evil I abhor, and have
No fear of God before my eyes;
Self-harden'd in my lost estate,
All sin I love, all good I hate.
.....

8. O God, regard my bitter cry,
I groan to be redeem'd from sin;
To Thee I lift my weeping eye,
Open Thine arms and take me in;
To Thee my labouring soul I bow;
Require it, O require it now.

9. I know it is not now renew'd,
I am not fit Thy face to see,
But trust the virtue of Thy blood
In my last hour shall work on me
Some miracle of grace unknown,
Without a miracle undone.[104]

[Hymn 2]
Hebrews 2: 10

1. Could sufferings heighten or complete
His full essential holiness?
No; but they made our Captain meet
To save a lost, apostate race:
His sufferings laid the ransom down,
And bought mine everlasting crown.

2. His death completes the sacrifice,
And shows the consecrated way,
That we might on His cross arise,
By suffering, as by works, obey,
And while we all His pangs endure,
Expect His blood to make us pure.

3. Thy passion, Lord, and not our own,
Doth peace and purity impart;
Thy blood which did for sin atone,
Writes pardon on the sprinkled heart,
And by the Spirit of faith applied,
It perfects all the crucified.

4. Who daily bleed and die with Thee,
Thou dost with perfect patience bless,
Redeem'd from all iniquity,
Restored to all the life of grace,
And by this narrow way alone,
Thou lead'st us to Thy glorious throne.[105]

[Hymn 3]
A Welcome to the Cross

1. All hail the Saviour's hallow'd cross,
By which I daily die within!
All things for Thee I count but loss:
Enter my soul, and work out sin;
Here let Thy mortal virtue move,
And crucify my creature-love.

2. Wither my strength, destroy my will,
Stain all the glory of my pride,
My appetites and passions kill,
Be to my whole of self applied,
Implunge me in the depth beneath,
And speak to all my nature death.

3. O that I now with all could part,
Cut off my hand, pluck out the eye!
Jesus, Thou greater than my heart,
Thine efficacious death apply;
Now for Thyself prepare the way;
Breathe, and the sinful *Adam* slay.

4. Thou know'st what keeps me out of Thee,
Naked I in Thine eyes appear:
Reveal the thing I would not see,
The'accursed thing that harbours here;
O, tear it hence, although the smart,
The killing anguish break my heart.

5. Thou seest, alas! I am not dead,
My nature's life in me is whole;
Again the rebel lifts his head,
And self bears down my struggling soul;
This thorn, I feel it in my side,
The'unconquerable strength of pride.

6. Still do I live, not Christ, but I;
The inbred sin I groan to bear;
Jesu, with Thee I long to die,
The suffering of Thy cross to share,
Sweet fellowship with Thee to have:
Bury me Saviour, in Thy grave.

7. There let me lay my burden down
In sweet forgetfulness of care:
The cross shall bring me to the crown,
The dead Thy praises shall declare;
When all renew'd in love I shine,
Partaker of a life Divine.[106]

Notes

1. Sarah Ryan to Mrs. Barker, [nd] Letters, 6 in "Further Account of Mrs. Ryan." MA 24.3, F/T.

2. "Life of Mrs. Ryan," 74. MA 24.1. F/T.

3. "Life of Mrs. Ryan," 8. MA 24.1. F/T.

4. Methodists did not use the term *Busskampf*, but it is a convenient term for an experience they described in a variety of phrases, including "groaning for redemption," "mourning for sin," being "awakened" and being "convicted of sin."

5. Sermon 4: 1 John 3: 14. Newport, ed., *Sermons*, 137–45.

6. Sermon 4: 1. Newport, ed., *Sermons*, 137.

7. Sermon 4: 1. Newport, ed., *Sermons*, 144–45.

8. *HSP* (1742): "Groaning for Redemption, Part IV." *PW* 2: 165. Eight verses in all.

9. Two series of hymns on "Groaning for Redemption" can be found in *PW* 2: 126–33, 159–65. See also *HSP* (1749): "For One Convinced of Unbelief, Hymns I–X." *PW* 4: 322–34.

10. Saul committed suicide after being defeated in battle. See 1 Samuel 31: 4.

11. Mrs. Margaret Austin to Charles Wesley, 19 May 1740. EMV 1.

12. For many examples taken from letters to Charles Wesley, see Hindmarsh, *The Evangelical Conversion* Narrative, 139–59.

13. Hindmarsh, *The Evangelical Conversion Narrative*, 139.

14. These verses were originally published by Charles Wesley as part of a lengthy hymn on Jeremiah 17: 9. The longer hymn clearly deals with the experience of mourning over sin and John published it in his *Collection of Hymns for the Use of the People Called Methodists* (1780) in the section "For Mourners Brought to the Birth." *BEW* 7: 271.

15. For examples, see Mrs. Platt to Charles Wesley, 20 Sept. 1738. EMV 10; Elizabeth Pratt to Charles Wesley, 12 Apr. 1740. EMV 11; Mary Ramsay to Charles Wesley, 4 June 1740. EMV 14.

16. "Life of Sarah Ryan," 28–29. MA 24.1, F/T.

17. Chilcote, ed., *Her Own Story*, 156. Taft was quoting from one of Wesley's "Redemption Hymns," *PW* 7: 81.

18. *PW* 2: 95. Wesley links the cross and the crown throughout his hymns. A few examples include *PW* 1: 330, 3: 324, 4: 44, 5: 70, 5: 209, 10: 212, 10: 335, 11: 38, 11: 86, 12: 37, 12: 54, 12: 84, 13: 47.

19. *SHSPHS* (1762): "Mark 10: 38." *PW* 11: 36.

20. Emphasis mine.

21. Another obvious use of "cup" with reference to Christ's suffering and God's judgment is in Matthew 26: 39, describing Jesus in the garden of Gethsemane before his arrest. "And he went a little further, and fell on his face, and prayed, saying, O my Father, if it be possible, let this cup pass from me: nevertheless not as I will, but as thou wilt."

22. *SHSPHS* (1762): "John 1: 37." *PW* 11: 327–28.

23. For example, Isaiah 53: 3.

24. Sarah Ryan to Mrs. Barker, [nd] Letters, 4 in "Further Account of Mrs. Ryan." MA 24.3, F/T.

25. Ann Martin to Charles Wesley, 1740. EMV 4.

26. Mrs. Susanna Designe to John Wesley, 31 Dec. 1741. Colman Collection.

27. Margaret Davidson to [Mrs. Agnes Smyth?], 8 Jan. 1777. Chilcote, ed., *Her Own Story*, 207.

28. Abraham Jones to John Wesley, 12 Dec. 1742. Colman Collection.

29. Thompson, *The Making of the English Working Class*, 406.

30. For a balanced critique of Thompson's arguments, see Hempton and Walsh, "E. P. Thompson and Methodism," 99–120.

31. Thompson, *The Making of the English Working Class*, 409.

32. Thompson, *The Making of the English Working Class*, 406.

33. John H. Wigger, *Taking Heaven by Storm: Methodism and the Rise of Popular Christianity in America* (New York, Oxford: Oxford University Press, 1998), 19.

34. See Rack, *Reasonable Enthusiast*, 334; Newport, ed., *Sermons*, 334–40.

35. Sermon 1: Philippians 3: 13–14. Newport, ed., *Sermons*, 101.

36. John Wesley was reading Taylor and a Kempis in 1725, and probably began reading Law's works in 1730. Rack, *Reasonable Enthusiast*, 73–74, 396.

37. Rack, *Reasonable Enthusiast*, 73.

38. *HSP* (1739): "Free Grace." *PW* 1: 106.

39. Sermon 5: Titus 3: 8. Newport, ed., *Sermons*, 163–64.

40. See my discussion of Charles Wesley's doctrine of atonement in Chapter Three.

41. Sermon 5: Titus 3: 8. Newport, ed., *Sermons*, 164–65.

42. Issues relating to the doctrine of sanctification were tangentially involved in the Wesleys' split with the Moravians in 1740 and at the heart of the dispute with Calvinist Evangelicals that exploded in 1770. Rack provides a detailed analysis of these disputes in *Reasonable Enthusiast*, 202–7, 450–61.

43. For John Wesley's changing understanding of perfection, see Rack, *Reasonable Enthusiast*, 395–401.

44. Rack, *Reasonable Enthusiast*, 398–99.

45. For Charles Wesley's view of perfection, see Tyson, ed., *Charles Wesley*, 39–40, 360–97.

46. *SHSPHS* (1762): "Hebrews 6: 1." *PW* 13: 133.

47. John Wesley to Charles Wesley, 9 July 1764. Tyson, ed., *Charles Wesley*, 384.

48. For example, *PW* 1: 262–65, 2: 159–66, 2: 196–97, 4: 453–54, 10: 14–15.

49. Rack, *Reasonable Enthusiast*, 398–99.

50. Mack, "Religious Dissenters in Enlightenment England," 19.

51. *SHSPHS* (1762): "Hebrews 12: 10." *PW* 13: 157–58.

52. *HSP* (1749): "In Temptation, Hymn 12." *PW* 4: 478–79.

53. Charles Wesley to Sarah Gwynne, 12 Aug. 1748. DDWES 4/96. For examples of Methodists desiring sanctification, see Katherine Gilbert to Charles Wesley, 1740. EMV 6; Samuel Webb to Charles Wesley, 20 Nov. 1741. EMV 18; Thomas Cooper to Charles Wesley, 1741. EMV 16; William Barber to Charles Wesley, 1741. EMV 20.

54. *HSP* (1742): "For a Sick Friend." *PW* 2: 216.

55. *SHSPHS* (1762): "Hebrews 2: 10 (ii)." *PW* 13: 121.

56. *HSP* (1749): "Hymns for Believers. Hymn 31." *PW* 5: 50.

57. Elizabeth Sais to Charles Wesley, May 1742. EMV 126.

58. Susanna Designe to John Wesley, 31 Dec. 1741, Colman Collection.

59. Mary Maddern to Charles Wesley, 29 June 1762. EMV 105.

60. Luke 23: 29 ("One of the malefactors, which were hanged, railed on him"). *UP* 2: 203.

61. See *Hymns for Children* (1763): "Of Hell." *PW* 6: 377–78.

62. See, for example, *PW* 9: 233–34, 9: 356, 9: 391, 9: 425, 10: 51–52.

63. Amato, *Victims and Values*, 44–63; Porter, "Pain and Suffering," 2: 1584–87.

64. Amato, *Victims and Values*, 50–51.

65. Amato, *Victims and Values*, 59.

66. Amato, *Victims and Values*, 61–63.

67. Key verses on suffering include Mark 8: 34b, Hebrews 12: 6–8, 1 Peter 1: 6–7, 2 Corinthians 4: 17, Romans 5: 3–5b.

68. Tyson, ed., *Charles Wesley*, 43.

69. For a discussion of this theme in medieval mysticism, see Denys Turner, *The Darkness of God: Negativity in Christian Mysticism* (Cambridge: Cambridge University Press, 1995).

70. "Mark 2: 19–20." *UP* 2: 52.

71. For example, *PW* 1: 330–32, 9: 239, 10: 14, 10: 51, 10: 76.

72. For example, *PW* 8: 408, 13: 69–70, 13: 127–28, 13: 129–31.

73. John Wesley, "On Self-Denial." Outler, ed., *Sermons II*, vol. 2, *BEW*, 244.

74. Wesley, "On Self-Denial," 243.

75. John Wesley, "Heaviness through Manifold Temptations." Outler, ed., *Sermons II*, vol. 2, *BEW*, 233.

76. John Wesley, "The Wilderness State." Outler, ed., *Sermons II*, vol. 2, *BEW*, 219.

77. Wesley, "Heaviness through Manifold Temptations," 234–35.

78. Wesley, "The Wilderness State," 208.

79. Wesley, "The Wilderness State," 212–13.

80. Wesley, "The Wilderness State," 219.

81. *SHSPS* (1762): "Hebrews 12: 8." *PW* 13: 156–57.

82. *PW* 13: 157.

83. Mon., 15 Dec. 1788. Ward and Heitzenrater, eds., *Journal and Diaries VII (1787–91)*, vol. 24, *BEW*, 117.

84. For another example of John's emphasis on "cheerfulness" as an appropriate emotion for the Christian, see his discussion of "that cheerfulness which is highly proper at a Christian meal" in his sermon "The More Excellent Way." Albert C. Outler, ed., *Sermons III*, vol. 3, *BEW* (Nashville: Abingdon, 1984), 262–67.

85. Thompson, *The Making of the English Working Class*, 417. Hempton and Walsh comment on the problematic nature of this portrayal of Methodism in "E. P. Thompson and Methodism," 108.

86. When John published his *A Collection of Hymns for the Use of the People Called Methodists*, the section "For Believers Suffering" contained ten hymns, eight of which were written by Charles Wesley. Only one of the hymns contains an extended comparison between the suffering of Christ and the suffering of believers. It includes the statement, addressed to Christ, that believers "must all Thy state of suffering share." Hildebrandt and Beckerlegge, eds., *A Collection of Hymns for the Use of the People called Methodists*, vol. 7, *BEW*, 476–78.

87. Hempton and Walsh, "E.P. Thompson and Methodism," 108.

88. "Further Account of Mrs. Ryan," 16. MA 24.3. F/T. Emphasis in original.

89. Letters, 20 in "Further Account of Mrs. Ryan," MA 24.3. F/T.

90. "Further Account of Mrs. Ryan," 24. MA 24.3. F/T.

91. See Susanna Designe to Charles Wesley, 8 Apr. 1742. CW Box; Joseph Carter to Charles Wesley, Nov. 1741. EMV 17; Wesley, EMV 16.

92. An interesting comparison can be made in this regard between the descriptions given by two Methodist women of sanctification. Mrs. Ann Ray, writing to Elizabeth Hurrell, wrote of the value of "crosses, trials or temptations" in bringing about submission to Christ, but mentioned it as only one of various means to holiness. Hester Ann Rogers encouraged a correspondent to look for perfection, not through suffering but through faith. Once such a state was received, she contended, there might be "a degree of heaviness" at times, but not for long. See Chilcote, ed., *Her Own Story*, 199–202 and 10–13.

93. A. Gregory Schneider, *The Way of the Cross Leads Home: The Domestication of American Methodism* (Bloomington and Indianapolis: Indiana University Press, 1993), 54.

94. Schneider, *The Way of the Cross Leads Home*.

95. "Life of Mrs. Ryan," 23. MA 24.1. F/T. Quoted in Mack, "Religious Dissenters in Enlightenment England," 12.

96. "Life of Mrs. Ryan," 32–33. MA 24.1. F/T.

97. The Methodist Conference had agreed upon rubrics controlling the preaching of women within Methodist structures in 1803. Chilcote, ed., *Her Own Story*, 278.

98. Chilcote, ed., *Her Own Story*, 171.

99. John Wesley to Mary Bishop, 1 Apr. 1773. Chilcote, ed., *Her Own Story*, 148.

100. For a brief account of Dorothy Ripley's life, see Chilcote, ed., *Her Own Story*, 122–23, 30–31.

101. Dorothy Ripley, "An Account of the Extraordinary Conversion and Religious Experience of Dorothy Ripley," in Chilcote, ed., *Her Own Story*, 136. Ripley's use of the word "if" suggests that she did not accept Charles Wesley's insistence on the necessity of great suffering, but she clearly saw such suffering as having spiritual benefit.

102. Mack, "Religious Dissenters in Enlightenment England," 8–9.

103. Schneider argues convincingly that "the way of the cross" initially subverted both the patriarchy and the honor culture of the American South but that it was eventually domesticated in ways that limited opportunities for women. See Schneider, *The Way of the Cross Leads Home*, 59–77. For a broader overview of the expanding and contracting of opportunities for women in Methodism, see Hempton, *Methodism*, 137–50.

104. *HSP* (1942): "Groaning for Redemption, Part I." *PW* 2: 159–60.

105. *SHSPS* (1762): "Hebrews 2: 10 (II)." *PW* 13: 119–21.

106. *HSP* (1742): "A Welcome to the Cross." *PW* 2: 94–95.

Chapter Five

Suffering and the Sanctified Self

In early December 1753, Charles Wesley traveled from his home in Bristol to London, where his brother John lay dangerously ill. Charles left behind him his wife, Sally, and their first child, Jacky. Three days after his arrival in London, he recorded in his journal a conversation with some Methodist laywomen, who had recommended that Sally be inoculated against smallpox:

> I answered, that I left everyone to his own conscience; but, for my part, I looked upon it as taking the matter out of God's hands; and I should choose, if it depended on me, to trust her entirely to Him.[1]

Returning to his accommodation that afternoon, Charles received word that Sally had been taken ill with smallpox of the most dangerous and painful kind. He raced back to Bristol. Upon arrival, he found:

> my dearest friend on a restless bed of pain, loaded with the worst kind of the disease... The whole head faint, and the whole heart sick! From the crown of the head to the soles of her feet there is no soundness. Yet, under her sorest burthen, she blessed God that she had not been inoculated, receiving the disease as immediately sent from Him. I found the door of prayer wide open, and entirely acquiesced in the divine will.[2]

For the next five days, he attended her sickbed and watched her grow worse and worse, then slowly better. With Sally fully recovered he left Bristol again, only for their infant son, Jacky, to catch the smallpox. Before Charles could return home, Jacky had died.

Charles Wesley's account of this crisis demonstrates his understanding of suffering as spiritual drama: the decision with regard to inoculation is understood as a matter of faith; his description of Sally's sufferings is couched in biblical language; his concern is primarily with the moral aspect of his wife's (and his own) conduct in the face of the disease. In Wesley's account the disease itself, as well as the responses of those affected by it, are loaded with spiritual meanings. This account makes sense within the broader contours of his understanding of human suffering, as demonstrated in the previous chapter. If Christian suffering was an essential part of God's work in the individual, an attack of smallpox could take on profound spiritual meaning. Understanding such meanings allowed the sufferer to respond in appropriate ways: Sally's terrible agony could be received with resignation, "as immediately sent from Him," and her husband could "entirely acquiesce in the divine will."

Wesley clearly presented his and Sally's responses to suffering as exemplary, which raises the question: how could such attitudes to suffering be developed? How could the devout individual learn to discern in his or her own experience of suffering such profound spiritual meanings? How could the appropriate response of submission be cultivated in the face of the overwhelming pain of the body or mind? Wesley's hymns clearly acted as aids to developing such responses. Many of the hymns were designed to be used with regard to specific experiences of suffering: as tools for remembering past suffering, managing present suffering or preparing for future suffering in ways that were spiritually beneficial. These hymns provided early Methodists with a model of how to suffer in particular situations, determining what could legitimately be experienced as suffering and what responses should be offered to such experiences. Wesley's construction of individual experiences of suffering intersects at many points with broader discourses within eighteenth-century English culture.

Sanctifying Smallpox

Wesley's response to his wife's experience of smallpox provides a useful starting point for this analysis. Some years after Sally's bout of smallpox, Wesley published two hymns titled "Thanksgiving After Recovery from the Small-pox."[3] While these hymns may not refer specifically to Sally's recovery, they were written after her illness and recovery and surely drew upon this experience. Read within the context of Sally's experience, these hymns provide insight into the process of interpreting an individual experience of suffering for spiritual benefit. For example, the second of the two hymns echoes the language used in Wesley's journal account, but constructs the experience somewhat differently.

> 1. Sing to the Prince of life and peace
> Let every tongue *my* Saviour bless
> So strong to help in danger's hour,
> So present in His healing power,
> And from the margin of the grave
> So good a dying worm to save.
>
> 2. Can I forget the solemn day
> When grappling with my foe I lay?
> O'er my weak flesh from foot to head
> The loathsome leprosy was spread,
> The foulest plague our race can feel,
> The deadliest fruit of sin and hell.

3. The poison boil'd in every vein,
The fire broke out in raging pain,
I sunk oppress'd through all my powers,
With bruises, wounds and putrid sores,
My body rack'd in every part,
And sick to death my fainting heart.

4. Jesus beheld my last distress,
And turn'd the current of disease,
He stopp'd my spirit on the wing,
And chased away the grisly king;
His wonder-working arm I own,
And give the praise to God alone.

5. He in the kind physician came,
(Bow all to Jesus' balmy name!)
Amidst my weeping friends He stood,
And mix'd the cordial with His blood,
Display'd His dead-reviving art,
And pour'd His life into my heart.

6. Brought from the gates of death, I give
My life to Him by whom I live;
Raised from a restless bed of pain,
I render Him my strength again,
And only wait to prove His grace,
And only breathe to breathe His praise.[4]

This hymn is concerned with memory: the memory of suffering, and recovering from, smallpox. As the second verse asks: "Can I forget the solemn day/ when grappling with my foe I lay?" This memory is constructed by means of a narrative that provides the reader or singer of this hymn with a spiritual or theological interpretation of his or her experience. The basic thrust of this narrative is summarized in the first verse, where Christ is to be praised for being "So strong to help in danger's hour/ So present in his healing power." As these lines indicate, this hymn tells the story of a rescue from death. Verses two to five describe the rescue in more detail, with verses two and three giving a description of the experience of having smallpox, and verses four and five describing the recovery from smallpox.

In verse two, smallpox is personalized as a "foe" against whom the individual struggles, and this introduces a theme of battle that continues through the hymn. In the contemporary context, this is not an original metaphor for understanding smallpox, as a number of poems from Wesley's time compared the experience of smallpox with battle.[5] Smallpox is also compared here to afflictions with particular biblical significance – the plagues and leprosy. Both are connected in biblical thought with uncleanness and the judgment of God, and there is a long history of the exploration and reinforcement of these connections in the medieval and early modern experience of leprosy and the plague.[6] But smallpox, the hymn claims, is "the *foulest* plague our race can feel,/ the *deadliest* fruit of sin and hell."

Smallpox is explained not simply as a physical struggle, but as a spiritual and theological one. Within this framing, verse three gives a vivid and convincing picture of the physical realities of the experience, probably reflecting Wesley's long vigil beside his wife's sickbed. The boiling veins, the "raging pain," the "bruises, wounds and putrid sores" heighten the memory of how terrible the suffering was. The language of "oppression" reinforces the idea that this suffering represents a personal attack. The literary effect of this portrayal of smallpox is to produce the dramatic effect of verses four and five. Here God enters the story, not as the one who brings disease, but as the one who saves from disease. Jesus appears on the battlefield triumphantly: he "turn'd" the current of disease, he "stopp'd my spirit on the wing," he "chased away" the grisly King Death.

Just as the memory of the disease has been constructed in spiritual terms, so in the following verses the memory of recovery is constructed in spiritual terms. The doctor, the weeping friends and the medicine are all portrayed as means by which Jesus has personally acted in the situation to bring about physical healing. A feature of smallpox was that the sufferer usually remained conscious.[7] Survivors of smallpox might well remember the presence of anxious friends, the arrival of the doctor and the administration of medicines. This hymn gives these memories profound significance within the wider story of the rescue. The appropriate response to this delivery, as the final verse concludes, is overwhelming gratitude and total commitment to Christ.

When read within the context of the many contemporary poetic accounts of smallpox, this hymn emerges as unusual in an important regard. By the mid-eighteenth century, smallpox was the leading infectious cause of premature death in England.[8] Not surprisingly, numerous contemporary poets explored the horrors of the disease. Most of these poets, however, focused on the extent to which smallpox ravaged the human body, causing a terrible transformation through blistering and scarring.[9] Poems about smallpox survivors concentrated on the moral and emotional consequences of the scars that smallpox left behind.[10] This was particularly true for those poems that explored the experience of smallpox for young women.[11] In these poems, the suffering of smallpox was located as much in its aftermath as in the disease itself.

In Wesley's hymn, the physical transformation that smallpox caused is not mentioned, even though the disease left Sally Wesley terribly scarred.[12] The post-smallpox body, in this hymn, is defined not by disfigurement, but by total commitment to Christ: "I render Him my strength again…And only breathe to breathe His praise." While the suffering of the disease itself is emphasized as the context in which Christ delivers, the possibility of further suffering in the aftermath is ignored. The hymn thus defines what suffering may be considered legitimate. Physical pain is recognized as meaningful suffering in this hymn but, for the devout Methodist, the loss of beauty should not constitute suffering.

The pattern of the narrative in these verses – the dire situation of the individual followed by Christ's dramatic intervention and the resulting transformation of the individual's situation – clearly follows that of Methodist conversion narratives. Just as in such a narrative, here it is Christ's blood that is able to save, to bring the dead back to life. Just as in such a narrative, the appropriate ending is a proclamation of absolute gratitude and commitment. If a conversion narrative told the story of a life in which Christ intervened to bring salvation, a hymn such as this one tells the story of one episode in the individual's life that repeats and reinforces the broader pattern. The theological conviction that suffering brought sanctification is here expressed in the context of a bout of smallpox that brings about an increased spiritual commitment. The memory of terrible suffering is given meaning within this narrative of transformation.

A comparison between this hymn and the account of Sally Wesley's illness in Wesley's journal reveals two alternative responses to the same (or a similar) experience. In the journal account, written in the midst of the experience, Wesley framed Sally's suffering as the gift of a loving and omnipotent divine will, to be responded to with obedience and resignation. In the hymn, written once recovery was certain, his emphasis changed. Smallpox became a "foe" to be grappled with, an enemy that only Christ could conquer. While these different approaches may suggest certain tensions in Wesley's theology, particularly in regard to the appropriate agency of the individual, they also point to the flexibility of his approach. One experience of suffering could be imbued with layers of meaning.

The "Language of the Rod"

The key to understanding Wesley's approach in these hymns is found in his use of phrases such as "the language of the rod," as in a short hymn on Micah 6: 9.

Father, Thy kind design explain
In every scourge and cross,
What is the meaning of *this* pain,
This trouble, or *this* loss?
O might my heart distinctly hear
The language of the rod,
Answer Thy will, and always fear,
And always love my God.[13]

This hymn expresses Wesley's conviction that every "pain," "trouble" or "loss" had a distinct purpose in the life of the believer, and thus a particular meaning that the devout individual could discern. As was demonstrated in the previous chapter, he understood Christian suffering as a necessary part of the process of sanctification. Only those disciplined by the "cross" of suffering could receive the heavenly "crown." This hymn clearly displays such an understanding of suffering as a "scourge" and "cross" that fulfilled God's purposes. It further suggests, however, that in the specific situation of the individual, different sufferings contributed to sanctification in different ways. This hymn encourages the believer to perceive specific experiences of suffering as communications from God, each with a particular meaning that must be correctly interpreted and responded to for sanctification to continue. The conviction that suffering was redemptive (following Christ) led the believer to focus on his or her own life, to ensure that suffering accomplished its purpose.

The wider writings of John and Charles Wesley demonstrate the theological convictions that contributed to such an understanding of suffering. In particular, their understanding of the workings of providence contributed to a belief that at the most specific level, personal experiences were laden with spiritual meanings. John's sermon "On Divine Providence" emphasizes the control of God over each and every aspect of life. John argued that God is omnipotent, omniscient, omnipresent and all-loving: "He doeth whatsoever pleaseth him, in heaven and earth, and in the sea and all deep places: And we cannot doubt of his exerting all his power, as in sustaining, so in governing, all that he has made."[14] Having argued for God's overarching control of all things, John then went on to distinguish between the concern that God has for "real Christians" and others. God loves all people, John contended, even "Mahometans and Heathens": "The Lord is loving unto every man, and his mercy is over all his works."[15] Those who serve him truly, however, are the particular object of his care.

> He sees their souls and their bodies; he takes particular notice of all their tempers, desires and thoughts, all their words and actions. He marks all their sufferings, inward and outward, and the source whence they arise... Nothing relative to these is too great, nothing too little, for His attention.[16]

As God is concerned for the details of human life, so he controls and acts through these details, willingly deviating from the "general laws" of creation in order to rescue or bless his people. He uses even the actions of sinful people to bring about good for those who trust him.

In explaining providence in these terms, John was consciously affirming a traditional understanding of providence over and against more contemporary interpretations. Seventeenth-century Calvinists, both in and out of the Church of England, had explained God's work in the world in similar terms, taking their interpretative framework from John Calvin himself.[17] Like John Wesley, these Calvinists distinguished between God's universal providence in sustaining the world and his "particular" care for Christians while also asserting that God controlled every aspect of creation. In affirming this view, John explicitly rejected the increasingly popular notion of "general" Providence, which held that God acted in the world only through the laws of nature. Newtonian physics, along with the other discoveries of seventeenth- and early eighteenth-century natural philosophers, seemed to provide increasing support for the arguments of those who opposed the idea of a God more intimately involved in the workings of the universe.[18] John argued, however, that this concept of "general Providence" was "stark, staring nonsense as any man of sense ought to be utterly ashamed of."[19]

While there is no record of Charles explaining the theology of providence in such detail, he appears to have shared John's understanding. He copied out and repeatedly preached an early sermon of John's, which argued that: "All [God's] providences, be they mild or severe, point at no other end than this. They are all designed either to wean us from what is not, or to unite us to what is worthy [of] our affection."[20] In his journal, Charles attributed diverse events to the workings of providence: a timely warning against a landslide; the escape of a "poor drunkard" during the collapse of his house; the broken leg of a boy who caused disturbances during a Methodist meeting; guidance through strange terrain; the reading of particularly meaningful Scripture and delivery from death (for Charles and his attackers) during an ambush.[21] Belief in an all-powerful and all-loving God directing every event of life encouraged close attention to the events of one's own life as a source of evidence as to God's purposes.

This interpretation applied equally to events on a broader scale. This is demonstrated in a number of hymns that Wesley wrote "For the Nation," in 1782. For example, in "Thanksgiving for the success of the Gospel in America," Wesley portrays the nation as experiencing "desolating judgments" that work to bring about salvation.

1. Glory to our redeeming Lord,
Whose kingdom over all presides,
While in the chariot of the word,
And on the whirlwind's wings He rides.

2. Nothing His rapid course can stay,
Or stop His government's increase;
Earthquakes and plagues prepare His way,
Wars usher in the Prince of peace.

3. Rebellions, massacres and blood
On every side as water shed,
Are suffer'd by a righteous God,
That happier days may then succeed.

4. Even now His word doth swiftly run,
And saving knowledge multiplies,
And still His gracious work goes on,
And still His temple's walls arise.
...

7. In love He doth His sons chastise,
His desolating judgments send!
Judgments are mercies in disguise,
And all in man's salvation end.[22]

As this hymn makes clear, sinful actions such as "rebellions" and "massacres" are "suffer'd" by God in order to accomplish his loving purposes. Such a view encouraged Methodists to interpret events of national significance, such as wars, invasion or earthquakes, within the same theological framework they applied to more individual experiences. When encountering such affliction, the nation must examine its collective conscience, repent of sin and submit to God's rule.[23]

The significance given to suffering in the process of sanctification, in combination with the Wesleys' theology of providence, meant that it was very important for the believer to examine each experience of suffering and consider its meaning. The broad sanctifying purposes of suffering could be understood by recognizing the pattern of Christ's life: the cross that led to the crown. As Charles preached:

> For to those who have ears to hear, every loss, especially of what was nearest and dearest to them, speaks as clearly as if it were an articulate voice from heaven, "Little children, keep yourselves from idols." Every pain cries aloud, "Love not the world, neither the things of the world."[24]

The exact purposes of a particular experience of suffering – the particular "idol" that the experience was designed to destroy – could only be understood by prayer, attention to Scripture and to one's own life. Suffering was a language that the believer must interpret by asking, "What is the meaning of *this* pain, *this* trouble or *this* loss?"

The letters written to Charles Wesley show Methodist men and women attempting exactly this task of interpretation, a process often fraught with anxiety. Elizabeth Marriot recorded her mother's anxious words: "I often think wherefore my body is so afflicted; sometimes I think it is a token for good that the Lord will save me, and therefore my sin has its punishment here; at other times I fear it is only an earnest of eternal misery." Elizabeth encouraged her mother "to believe it was a token of his willingness to receive her after all she had done."[25] A Methodist named Mary Guy described her physical sufferings to Charles and concluded confidently: "I know this affliction is a merciful chastisement from God to bring me more to myself, and not forget him which is my earnest prayer."[26] For another writer, however, the dying agonies of her brother were troubling: "His last conflicts caused great uneasiness in me, that he that bore all his pain with that patient resignation should be so assaulted."[27]

For affliction to be of spiritual benefit, it must not only be interpreted correctly, but also responded to appropriately, as Charles and Sally exemplified in their time of trial. This was often no easy task. John Henderson described the painful cramps in his throat, stomach and limbs and concluded: "But of what use is precious pain, unless suffered in silence and felt as good?"[28] Ann Davis confessed:

> [T]here is times that I think I may say I am thankful for the rod and count it an honour to be admitted to taste of his cup but alas those happy moments are short and I sink again beneath the Cross which lies heavy and long upon my weary back.[29]

Mary Purnell described an ill sister: "When she was first taken, she could rejoice in suffering but now is out of all patience and sometimes wishes she was in hell that she might now the end of her misery."[30] As these letters suggest, terrible pain could challenge the best of intentions

For suffering to do its work in the life of the believer, therefore, the experience must be understood and responded to appropriately. As was suggested in the previous chapter, this task of interpreting and responding to suffering was not simply a matter of passive acceptance.[31] In the case of suffering resulting from sickness, Methodists were encouraged to diagnose their illness and actively seek healing through the use of medicine and other cures.[32] Orthodox Christian theology emphasized the value of the body and the Christian duty to care for it through all proper means.[33] In the preface to his book of *Primitive Physic,* John Wesley assured his readers that God provided health-giving food, doctors and medicine to "soften the evils of life, and prevent in part the sickness and pain to which we are continually exposed."[34] Charles wrote a "Physician's Hymn," which represented the perspective of the Christian doctor.

4. The friendly properties that flow,
Through nature's various works, I know
The Fountain whence they came;
And every plant, and every flower
Medicinal derives its power
From Jesu's balmy name.

5. Confiding in that name alone,
Jesus, I in Thy work go on,
To tend the sick and poor,
Dispenser of Thy medicines I;
But Thou the blessing must supply,
But Thou must give the cure.

6. For this I humbly wait on Thee;
The servant of Thy servants see
Devoted to Thy will,
Determined in Thy steps to go,
And help the sickly sons of woe,
Who groan Thy help to feel.

7. Afflicted by Thy gracious hand,
They now may justly all demand
My instrumental care;
Thy patients, Lord, shall still be mine;
And to my weak attempts I join
My strong effectual prayer.[35]

As this hymn demonstrates, Wesley interpreted the healing power of medicine through an evangelical emphasis on "Jesu's balmy name." The sick were God's patients and the physician merely his instrument. The experience of being restored to health reflected the experience of conversion, in which God graciously rescued the undeserving. The process of diagnosing and treating illness was thus placed in a theological context that gave it spiritual significance, requiring careful discernment.

The need for discernment can be seen in Wesley's account of his wife's smallpox: he represents inoculation as "taking the matter out of God's hands." But he was happy to make use of doctors and medicine in her treatment: his hymn on smallpox states that Jesus "in the kind physician came." Another Methodist convert, Taverner Wallis, wrote in his conversion narrative that after making spiritual progress for a time:

> I fell again, occasioned by taking too much care of my health and studying physic and being absent from under the Word, so that I thought the kingdom of heaven consisted in meats and drinks and trusted much in the means.[36]

Again, Wallis used a biblical quote, from Romans 14: 12, and the theologically laden term "means," to portray his experience of using medicine as part of a broader spiritual drama in which careful discernment was required.

While Wesley clearly saw the diagnosis and treatment of physical illness as spiritually significant, very few of his hymns focus on this process. Instead, hundreds of the hymns address the central issue that concerned Wesley and his fellow Methodists: how could suffering of all kinds be received for the spiritual benefit that God intended? A typical example is the first of a series entitled "For One in Pain" (see Hymn 1), which begins.

> 1. Pain, my old companion pain,
> Seldom parted from my side,
> Welcome to thy seat again,
> Here, if God permits, abide:
> Pledge of sure-approaching ease,
> Haste to stop my wretched breath,
> Rugged messenger of peace,
> Joyful harbinger of death.
>
> 2. Foe to nature as thou art,
> I embrace thee as my friend:
> Thou shalt bid my griefs depart,
> Bring me to my journey's end:
> Yes, I joyfully decay,
> Homeward through thy help I haste;
> Thou hast shook the house of clay;
> Surely it will fall at last.

This hymn aims to assist the singer or reader in achieving an attitude of resignation toward his or her pain. Pain is hailed in surprising terms, as "companion" and "friend." That this attitude to pain is counterintuitive is made explicit in verse two: "Foe to nature as thou art, I embrace thee as my friend." If pain is a "foe to nature," how can it be embraced?

The hymn encourages two attitudes that will produce a positive response to pain. Verses one to three emphasize pain as a welcome reminder of mortality: a "Joyful harbinger of death." Within the Methodist theological understanding, the death of the converted could be welcomed as their entrance into the joys of heaven.[37] Here and elsewhere, Wesley encourages such an attitude. Pain, as evidence of the body's "decay," is a "kind remembrancer" of death. The experience of suffering can be understood as an encouragement that suffering will one day be "no more."

The final two verses add a second element to this understanding by comparing physical pain with the spiritual pain of sin.

Who beneath thy pressure groan,
Chief of ills who reckon thee,
Sin, alas! they ne'er have known:
Sin is perfect misery.

In making this comparison, Wesley was not simply belittling the miseries of physical suffering. Rather, he was pointing to the role of this suffering: pain is a "salutory ill" that leads to freedom from sin in this life and, ultimately, to a "starry crown." Such a comparison draws on the consciousness of sinfulness that was encouraged in Methodists before and after conversion. The reader or singer of this hymn is thus encouraged to embrace his or her pain as both an encouraging reminder that heaven is near, and as a medicine against the far worse suffering of sinfulness. In understanding the "office" of this suffering and so accepting it, the reader or singer is appropriately thankful and resigned. Therefore, the experience of pain is "sanctified": it becomes a means of growth in personal holiness.

This hymn is clearly designed as a tool by which the believer can experience, interpret and respond to pain appropriately. That Wesley wrote so many hymns of this kind suggests that this was his central concern. The anxieties that early Methodists expressed suggest that it concerned many others within that culture. These anxieties are understandable, given the Methodist emphasis on self-control. As Mack has noted, Methodism showed a particular concern with self-mastery, the ability of the sanctified mind to shape the emotions and control the body.[38] As has been shown, Methodists understood such control not simply as an independent act of will, but as a divinely enabled submission of the self to God. "Self-submission" might be a more exact (though more clumsy!) term for the goal of Methodist practice. The centrality of this project for Methodists can be seen in the array of methods by which Methodists scrutinized and reformed their bodies, minds and emotions. These methods included "diet, exercise, mutual criticism and confession, autobiographical writing."[39] Wesley's hymns could be added to this list.

The concerns that individual Methodists expressed, about the need to rightly understand and control their responses to suffering, suggest that suffering could offer a particular threat to self-mastery and thus to spiritual safety and progress. This supports an understanding of suffering as a "total" or "engulfing" pain. This overwhelming experience offered an opportunity for total dependence on God and spiritual growth. But suffering could also lead men and women to think, feel or act in ways that were sinfully uncontrolled. Mack argues that this was a particular challenge for eighteenth-century women: "unlike men, who described the spiritual odyssey as a struggle to control anger, alcohol, or sexuality – the terrain on which women struggled for self-mastery was the terrain of bodily suffering."[40] The threat to "self-submission" and the opportunity for self-mastery that suffering represented help explain why Wesley devoted so many hymns to individual experiences of suffering. Within his theology of spiritual progress, each experience of suffering was an opportunity to move on toward sanctification, but it was also a possibility of being overwhelmed by suffering and falling away from God's grace.

While the hymn "For One in Pain" applies to the experience of physical suffering in general, other hymns offer responses for more specific experiences of suffering. To explore the complexity of these responses further, this chapter will consider hymns written for use in regard to four different kinds of suffering: persecution, public execution, childbirth and bereavement. Examining these different hymns reveals not only the ways in which particular experiences of suffering could be given meaning in a broader narrative of the Christian life, but also the ways in which such constructions compared to contemporary interpretations of these experiences.

Persecution

Charles Wesley, like many early English Methodists, had personal experience of persecution. Particularly in the first years of his itinerancy, his journal records many incidents of violent opposition that he and other Methodists encountered.[41] Wesley interpreted such opposition as evidence of the rightness of the Methodist cause and its similarity to the early, "primitive" church. While staying in Wednesbury, where the Methodists experienced significant persecution:

> I found the brethren assembled, standing fast in one mind and spirit, in nothing terrified by their adversaries... Never was I before in so primitive an assembly. We sang praises lustily, and with a good courage; and could all set our seal to the truth of our Lord's saying, "Blessed are they that are persecuted for righteousness' sake."[42]

As in this account, Wesley often mentioned singing hymns in the context of opposition, and he composed a number of hymns for those being persecuted.[43]

A typical hymn on persecution comes from a collection of such hymns, entitled *Hymns for Times of Trouble and Persecution*, published in 1745.

> 1. Lamb of God, we follow Thee,
> Willing as Thou art to be,
> Joyful in Thy steps to go,
> Suffering for Thy sake below.
>
> 2. Taking up our daily cross,
> Call'd to shame, and pain, and loss,
> Well contented to sustain
> All the rage of cruel men.
>
> 3. Who Thy lovely pattern knows
> Cannot force with force oppose,
> They that to Thy fold belong
> Dare not render wrong for wrong.

4. Bruised by the oppressor's hand,
Evil they will ne'er withstand,
All that follow Thee are meek.
Taught to turn the other cheek.

5. Jesu, in Thy gracious power
Lo! we meet the fiery hour,
Calm, dispassionate, resign'd,
Arm'd with all Thy patient mind.

6. After Thee with joy we come,
Sheep before our shearers dumb,
Answering not one angry word,
True disciples of our Lord.
...

8. Turn, almighty as Thou art,
Turn our persecutors' heart,
Let them to our faith be given,
Let us meet our foes in heaven.[44]

This hymn repeats Wesley's basic theological conviction that suffering in imitation of Christ is the lot of the Christian. Persecution is here included in this suffering, described as "our daily cross." This theme is used to emphasize that the appropriate response to such persecution is peaceful non-resistance: "All that follow Thee are meek,/ Taught to turn the other cheek." In the midst of the suffering of persecution, this hymn suggests, there is "joy" for the persecuted. In reading or singing this hymn, the persecuted exhort themselves to remain "Calm, dispassionate, resign'd," and so avoid repaying violence for violence. The hymn concludes with a prayer that the persecutors too might experience salvation. Other hymns in this series emphasize the "crown" of heavenly reward, and the joys of fellowship in suffering persecution together, as alternative incentives to remain resigned and non-violent in the face of assault.[45] They repeatedly emphasize an attitude of love and pity for the persecutor, rather than hatred or vengeance.[46]

For Methodists facing physical violence and social excommunication, the singing of such hymns provided a very personal exhortation to endure. These hymns encourage the reader or singer to be self-controlled: to resist the desire to retaliate, to avoid being overwhelmed by anger or hatred. Instead, these hymns suggest, the suffering of persecution can be overcome with joy.

On all the'affliction we look down,
The joy so far exceeds,
So bright, so weighty is the crown
It sets upon our heads.[47]

In these hymns, as in those "For one in Pain," self-control in the face of suffering is modeled and encouraged. Further, these hymns suggest that the true believer will be joyful in the face of suffering, understanding its true meanings.

This joy comes from identification with Christ in his suffering, which results in confidence that "the crown" of eternal life is assured.

Persecution is portrayed in these hymns as an experience of suffering that is straightforward to interpret. Its meanings are largely positive: persecution is clear evidence that the believer is following Christ faithfully and is assured of a heavenly reward. The suffering of the persecuted believer links very directly to the normative narrative of sanctifying suffering that Wesley promoted, making a joyful response relatively easy. Other Methodists certainly believed that persecution was a lesser challenge to faith than were other types of suffering. According to the Methodist leader John Fletcher:

> It is perhaps as hard to be racked with the gout, or to burn several days in a fever on a sick bed, as you or I may be forced to do, as to be for a few minutes with Shadrach and his companions in a burning furnace, or to feel for a fleeting moment the anguish of bruised flesh and a fractured skull with the triumphant martyr.[48]

In both Fletcher's depiction and Wesley's hymns, "triumph" is the expected experience of the persecuted one. The hymns only occasionally imply that such triumph might be difficult to attain, as in a hymn for the persecuted "at the Devizes":

> Thy weakest confessors defend,
> And let them on Thyself depend
> For help in their distress;
> Support, confirm the feeble mind,
> And keep them all on Thee reclined,
> And keep in perfect peace.[49]

Presumably, however, there were Methodists who were unable to muster such triumphant self-control at all, who responded to persecution by capitulating to their persecutors or who defended themselves with violence. These hymns give no voice to such a response.

Execution

In contrast to the hymns on persecution, Wesley also wrote a number of hymns for "condemned malefactors," those who had been sentenced to execution. As has been mentioned, following his conversion Wesley began a lifelong practice of visiting and preaching to those condemned to death.[50] While he had begun visiting those in prison many years earlier, his decision to preach to the condemned reflected his newfound belief in the possibility of last-minute conversion. His hymns display this conviction. In one of a series of *Prayers for Condemned Malefactors* written close to his death in the 1780s, Wesley wrote:

1. Justly by man condemn'd to die,
Jesus, the desperate sinner's Friend,
Out of the deep, regard our cry,
And O! let hope be in our end.

2. Suffering for ills which we have done,
The martyr's joy shall we require?
No: but we still for mercy groan,
And hope in final peace to' expire.

3. Before we gasp our latest breath,
Before we these vile bodies leave,
Remembering Thy own precious death,
Saviour, our parting souls receive.

4. Pluck us as brands out of the flame,
And wash'd in Thy atoning blood,
And saved through Thy almighty name,
Present our ransom'd souls to God.[51]

In this hymn, the suffering of those "justly" executed by the state is explicitly contrasted with the suffering of those who are martyred.[52] Those who are suffering as a result of "ills" that they have committed cannot expect the kind of triumphant joy that martyrs experience. The suffering of these "malefactors" is punishment, and the hymn clearly encourages them to accept it as such. Those condemned to die can, however, still hope for salvation, because of the possibility that Christ will remember his "own precious death" and forgive. The hymn thus draws the "malefactors'" attention to the state of their souls rather than their "vile bodies," and encourages a response of repentance and hope.

Wesley's other hymns for "condemned malefactors" represent the suffering of execution in similar ways, encouraging the condemned to penitently accept the sentence against them and direct their attention toward the life to come.[53] The experience of execution may not fit as comfortably into the ideal life narrative as the experience of persecution, but it is still easily given meaning within such a story. Last-minute conversions had great significance within early Methodism because they were a particular testimony to the amazing grace of God in justifying sinners who could in no way earn their salvation.[54] As John Walsh points out, the message of this grace "was dramatically represented by the attendance of Methodist preachers at public executions. Their presence at Tyburn represented… the accessibility of grace to the most despised and vulnerable of humankind."[55] The scriptural account of the repentant thief crucified next to Jesus, who was assured of a place in Paradise, provided a biblical trope for this experience that was particularly applicable to "condemned malefactors."[56] For these individuals, suffering was interpreted as an experience of judgment, the fear of which acted as a useful spur to consider the state of one's soul and the possibility of eternal suffering in hell. This is made even clearer in another hymn "For Condemned Malefactors": "Put them in fear; Thy wrath reveal;/ Shake o'er the opening mouth of hell,/ And scorch them with the flame."[57] Suffering for the malefactors was a matter of judgment, but it could be redemptive if it led them to repent and receive salvation.

This portrayal of execution is significant in the wider context of eighteenth-century debates over capital and corporal punishment.[58] Randall McGowen has argued that these debates involved a fundamental conflict over the meanings of the suffering body. Traditional attitudes to public execution gave primacy to the "body politic, a metaphor that spoke of a familiar set of relationships, of hierarchy and duty, and of a whole whose life was somehow directed by a purpose that no part could define."[59] This metaphor was repeatedly used in assize sermons and other addresses given on judicial occasions during the early eighteenth century. It conceptualized society as tightly connected through a web of relationships, but also as vulnerable to disease and corruption. As with the human body, such corruption might require drastic surgery to save the whole person. As McGowan points out, the most common metaphor used to describe public execution was that of "amputation." According to one eighteenth-century defender of execution: "The infected limb must be cut off, even in mercy, unless it be greater benefit to preserve one limb of the body, than all the rest."[60] While ideally this process of "amputation" would result in the repentance of the condemned individual, the primary concern was the well-being of the community. Within such an understanding of capital punishment, those who gazed upon the suffering bodies of the executed saw enacted the restoration of health to the body politic.

As has been mentioned earlier, the eighteenth century saw a growing resistance to such representations of capital punishment. Reformers contended that public execution was inhumane and ineffective, doing more harm than good to both criminals and society. These reformers reflected an alternative understanding of the suffering body, which gave primacy to the experience of the individual. In their understanding, "society was composed of separate bodies, of individuals who might be connected by interest and feeling rather than by a shared ceremonial life. The life of the individual was uniquely important, and sacrifice of the physical body would injure rather than heal the social body."[61] In this construction of society, sympathy and self-interest, rather than hierarchy and duty, were the forces that connected individuals to one another. Therefore, these reformers argued, the sight of a person being executed would not communicate complicated metaphorical meanings about the body politic; rather, it would overwhelm and distress the viewer.[62] This argument reflected not only an increasing emphasis on the power of sight, but also an understanding of the human body as powerfully representing individual identity.

Wesley's hymns for condemned malefactors were written throughout the period of these debates, and they reflect various aspects of these alternative understandings of public execution. Wesley affirmed the validity of capital punishment, encouraging the condemned to accept their execution as a just repayment for their crimes. He also affirmed the value of suffering for the individual, insofar as it warns of the dangers of hell that threaten. In this sense, Wesley's hymns represent a conservative understanding of execution, providing support for the claims of historians such as V. A. C. Gattrell and Peter Linebaugh, who have accused Methodism of contributing to the repressive culture of capital punishment in late eighteenth-century England.[63]

The primary focus of Wesley's hymns is not, however, on the social value of capital punishment, but on the individual experience of the condemned men and women. While defenders of public execution certainly hoped for a "good death" on the part of the executed, this was a secondary benefit of the punishment.[64] For Wesley, individual salvation was of central importance. In one hymn he did encourage the malefactors to warn those watching the "spectacle" of execution: "Now, now your evil ways forsake/ And 'scape the wrath to come."[65] This is, however, unusual. Even as Wesley affirmed the justice of capital punishment, he downplayed its traditional meanings in favor of a controversial emphasis on the urgent necessity of conversion. In focusing on the malefactor's experience in this way, Wesley opened the door to a more individualistic understanding of execution, one which undermined the traditional emphasis on the body politic.[66]

Childbirth

As has been argued, the emphasis in the hymns on suffering and the threat it posed to self-mastery could be particularly meaningful for women. While many (though certainly not all) of the Methodists who wrote to Wesley describing their struggles with physical suffering were women, few of Wesley's hymns imply that such mastery might be a particular matter of concern for women.[67] Mack suggests that Wesley was unusual among Methodist men in his attention to the spiritual threat posed by bodily pain.[68] While Wesley's emphasis on suffering could be described by a Victorian evangelical as inappropriately "feminine," the hymns assume that physical suffering is a challenge to Christians whatever their gender.[69] The significant exceptions to this are found in his series of hymns for women in "travail," which portray a powerful sense of the struggle for self-mastery that confronted women in labor.

One hymn from a series "For a Woman near the Time of her Travail" vividly depicts this struggle (see Hymn 2). In this depiction of childbirth, the greatest threat offered by childbirth is not the pain itself, or even death, but the spiritual danger that the pain represents. The possibility that suffering may overwhelm the woman's "patience" and "faith," and thus leave her "void" of God, is presented as her greatest terror. The hymn thus encourages the woman to pray, not for relief from pain or escape from death, but for spiritual sustenance. This sustenance is described specifically as the ability to control emotions: "Thy love shall all my griefs control,/ Thy love shall calm my fluttering soul." The assurance that God will provide this sustenance allows the woman to be "borne above" herself, to be "resign'd" to God's "bless'd will." The spiritual threat that childbirth represents is averted, and transformed into spiritual progress.

By singing or reading this hymn, the expectant mother placed her fear of suffering (a fear which, presumably, is a kind of suffering itself) within a theological context that gave it intense spiritual meaning. The hymn rehearses a narrative in which the woman is delivered from her fears and so masters them. This narrative again follows the familiar pattern of crisis, deliverance and transformation that was so important within Methodist culture. It places childbirth within the larger individual story of conversion and sanctification, which will end with an "infinite reward." The large number of similar hymns Wesley wrote for women before, during or after childbirth suggests that he understood childbirth as a particular challenge to women's self-control.[70] Writing to Sally during one of her pregnancies, he enquired, "Are you much in private prayer? Do you ever use my hymns for your condition?"[71]

Wesley's hymns also place the individual experience of childbirth within a broader narrative of human sinfulness and redemption. While, as has been discussed, Wesley understood all suffering as a consequence of sin, childbirth had particular meanings. In another hymn "For a Woman in Travail," Wesley affirmed that the pains of childbirth were ultimately a result of Eve's transgression in the garden of Eden. The hymn begins:

1. Jesus, we ask Thy promised aid;
Thou who for us a curse wast made,
The penalty extreme
Far from Thy chosen one remove,
And now the object of Thy love
From curse and death redeem.

2. First in the primitive offence
The curse she feels with quicker sense:
But, of a woman born,
Thou didst its utmost burden bear,
To make it fall more light on her,
And to a blessing turn.

3. With pity then the anguish see,
The fruits of sin endured by Thee,
Thou patient Man of Woe:
Thy sufferings past recall to mind,
Shorten in her Thy pangs behind,
And break the mortal blow.

4. In mercy mitigate her pain,
Her feeble fainting soul sustain
With comforts from above;
Strengthen, till all her pains are pass'd,
And let her every moment taste
The cordial of Thy love.

Because Eve was "First in the primitive offence," women feel "with quicker sense" the curse of suffering that sin has brought. This conviction is placed in the context of Wesley's overarching doctrine of recapitulation. The hymn explicitly parallels Christ's suffering to that of the woman in childbirth: the crucifixion is unusually described as the "bed" where Jesus "lay," and as his "travail."

Christ bore these sufferings to make Eve's curse "fall more light on her/ And to a blessing turn." Having endured these sufferings, Christ is also ready to sympathize with women in their ongoing sufferings. Childbirth thus becomes a micro-narrative of the broader theological pattern that Wesley saw at work, in which suffering as judgment is transformed by Christ's work into suffering as blessing.

As in the hymns describing the Passion, here the sight of Christ's suffering is depicted as central to the woman's experience. In verses five to seven, the sufferings of Christ are evoked through the description of his body:

> 5. Before her weary eyes display
> The bed where her Redeemer lay,
> A Lamb transfix'd and torn!
> The place Thou never canst forget,
> Where Thou hast paid our utmost debt,
> And all our sorrows borne.
>
> 6. O let Thy grief dry up her tears,
> And while Thy mangled form appears,
> Thy visage marr'd with blood,
> Let trouble, fear and torture cease,
> And all her happy soul confess
> Her Saviour and her God.
>
> 7. Victorious, with Thy cross in view,
> By Thy own travail bring her through
> The agonizing hour,
> A living monument of praise,
> A witness of redeeming grace,
> And love's eternal power.[72]

The sight of this suffering, which is conceptualized as a parallel experience of childbirth, empowers the woman to master herself. In this visual encounter, the sight of Jesus' pain overwhelms the woman's own feelings of pain, transforming "trouble, fear and torture" into happiness. This is an extraordinary victory of mind over body and emotions, achieved not simply by personal effort, but by the confronting vision of Christ's suffering. In the final verse, this victory is linked once again to the ongoing story of the individual's life, which will continue in appropriate "praise" for God's "grace."

This emphasis on seeing Christ's suffering appears only very occasionally in either the hymns on childbirth or the more general hymns on bodily suffering. While the depiction of Christ's suffering as a powerfully transformative sight echoes similar depictions in hymns about more general experiences of spiritual transformation, the emotions that this sight is described as evoking are quite different. In the context of personal suffering, awareness of Christ's suffering becomes a source of power to overcome: the woman in childbirth is described as "Victorious, with Thy cross in view." While it may seem counterintuitive to be empowered by a vision of weakness and suffering, here, as in the Passion hymns, the suffering of Christ is seen as the ultimate expression of God's love and compassion. In the period of intense crisis that extreme bodily pain produced, the sight of Christ's suffering was an overwhelming reminder of divine love. It was God's love as demonstrated in Christ's sufferings and death that ensured Christian suffering was meaningful and redemptive. Thus, where other hymns encourage the believer to reflect on the redemptive meanings of their suffering in a variety of ways, in a period of overwhelming pain and fear such as childbirth, a "sight" of Christ's suffering might be the means by which such meanings could be internalized.

The writings of Methodists reveal their attempts to imbue their sufferings with these meanings of love, through reflection on the sufferings of Christ. Sarah Ryan advised a friend:

> When you are in pain say, what pain my Lord hath born… If unkindly used, remember he was despised and rejected of men. Jesus loves you – love him again – cry for power to do so… tell him you will not let him go.[73]

Susanna Designe claimed, "It is nothing to suffer any affliction, either of body or mind, if there is but a small glimpse of Jesus."[74] On his deathbed, a young cabinetmaker received salvation, crying, "I see him, I see him – the Lamb, the Lamb."[75] Then, the Methodist attending him recorded,

> Sorrow and sighing fled away while he ate and drank of the bread and water of life… I asked him if he had any doubt or fear, he answered, "No, none at all" and said "I have no pain, I never had such pleasure in all my life. It runs all through me."

These accounts, and Wesley's hymns, suggested that Methodists could experience not just resignation, but joy in the midst of extreme physical suffering. This joy came from "a small glimpse of Jesus," an awareness of the suffering of Christ that reminded believers of his love and compassion. Methodism continued to hold out the possibility of such self-mastery in the face of suffering, and Methodist men and (especially) women continued to claim that they experienced such mastery on a daily basis.

Wesley's hymns on childbirth suggest that he perceived the struggle for self-control in the face of overwhelming physical pain to be an important but difficult process. This supports Mack's contention that the mastery of the self in bodily suffering was a significant element within early Methodist culture, and also that this struggle might have particular resonance for women who confronted the terrors of childbirth in eighteenth-century conditions. More broadly, it supports the contention that women's exposure to physical suffering had the potential to give them spiritual authority, if they overcame extraordinary pain. Wesley was also, however, concerned with emotional suffering. His hymns deal with emotional pains, such as the loss of loved ones through betrayal or bereavement, and they present these pains as equally a context for gaining self-mastery.

Death of Children

As has been mentioned, in 1754 Wesley's first child died of smallpox. Wesley expressed his grief at this loss in a number of hymns, written during the following ten years. Like the hymns on childbirth, these hymns represent the task of mastering oneself in the face of suffering as intensely difficult. Soon after Jacky's death Wesley wrote an eight-part sequence of hymns, which depicts an intense struggle to come to terms with his loss. The first hymn in the sequence is typical (see Hymn 3), beginning:

> 1. Dead! dead! the child I loved so well!
> Transported to the world above!
> I need no more my heart conceal:
> I never dared indulge my love:
> But may I not indulge my grief,
> And seek in tears a sad relief?

Wesley's moving lament for his son communicates clearly the struggle between "nature" and the duty to "bow… to the sovereign God." At the heart of this struggle was Wesley's love for his son, a love that was dangerous during Jacky's lifetime because it might "ensnare" his parents' "weak unguarded hearts." To "indulge" this love, the hymn suggests, would have been to tempt the jealous anger of God. If this understanding is shocking to the modern reader, for Wesley it apparently provided some comfort: Jacky had been delivered from the dangers of his parents' love and the evils of this world. They would eventually be reunited in heaven.

The effort to reach resignation is described and legitimized within this hymn: "But may I not indulge my grief/ And seek in tears a sad relief?" His "officious thoughts" turn repeatedly to his son's "winning gestures," which are described both to express Wesley's grief and to remind him of the spiritual danger that his love for his son represented. At the end of this hymn some level of resolution is depicted, but the struggle is repeated in the hymns that follow. Each hymn emphasizes that the death should be seen as a blessing, but "feeble flesh" and "nature" still grieve, as the sixth part of the sequence makes clear.

> 2. The child, of whom we seem bereaved,
> Whom feeble flesh would still deplore,
> Our heavenly Father hath received,
> And kindly bids us weep no more,
> But cheerfully His loan resign,
> And leave him in the arms Divine.
>
> 3. Father, we make Thy deed our own,
> Submissive to Thy wisest choice;
> Though nature give a parting groan,
> Our spirits *shall* in Thee rejoice,
> And thankfully at last approve
> Th' appointment of eternal love.[76]

If submission to God's will is ultimately achieved, these hymns suggest that it requires an enormous effort to achieve this state. This sequence of hymns provided, for its readers or singers, a model of the long, hard struggle to submit, and a tool for achieving this in their own lives. These hymns do not display the casual or triumphant attitude toward pain that appears in the hymns "For One in Pain" or the hymns for the persecuted. Rather, grief appears as a serious and nearly overwhelming challenge to the believer.

In presenting grief in this manner, these hymns present a startling contrast to a number of earlier hymns Wesley wrote on the death of a child. These were published in the second volume of the 1749 collection of *Hymns and Sacred Poems* and so written before Wesley himself had experienced such bereavement. The second hymn in a series "On the Death of a Child" is typical. The first two verses exemplify the tone of the whole:

1. Glory to that victorious grace,
Through which a worm can all things do!
I stand o'erwhelm'd with vast amaze,
And scarce believe the wonder true;
'Tis more than heart could e'er conceive,
I know my child is dead – and live!

2. Where is the passionate regret,
The fond complaint, and lingering smart?
Can I my sucking child forget,
So freely with my *Isaac* part,
So cheerfully my all resign,
And triumph in the will Divine![77]

This hymn, with its depiction of the parent "cheerfully" consigning their child to God's care without "passionate regret" or "lingering smart" obviously reflects an attitude that Wesley initially saw as desirable. While Wesley continued to write funeral hymns that depicted the death of adult believers as a matter for celebration, after the death of his own son he wrote no more hymns like this about children. It seems reasonable to conclude that his experience taught him that all grief was not so easily mastered.

Not surprisingly, letters from Methodists to Wesley suggest that the death of loved ones, particularly children, proved a difficult experience in which to find meaning or achieve resignation. Sally Wesley, writing to Charles to inform him that another of their sons, John James, had died at the age of seven months, called theology to her aid in achieving an exemplary attitude of resignation:

> It was a hard struggle before he could depart, he was dying all yesterday... he screamed three times about half an hour before he died, that he could be heard from nurse's parlour to the other side of the street. Not through guilt (that is my comfort) but through extreme pain. Perhaps were I of Calvin's opinion, I might have attributed it to a different cause, but glory be to a redeemer's love in declaring (for the consolation of distressed parents) 'that of such is the kingdom of heaven.'[78]

For the grieving mother, the meaning of her son's screams was crucial. If, as Calvin had argued, babies were inherently sinful and therefore potentially damned to hell, the screams could imply a guilty awareness of the coming judgment. A firm rejection of Calvin's opinion allowed Sally to affirm that her son was waiting for her in heaven.

In spite of such consolations, resignation was not easily achieved. In a letter describing the death of his wife, an acquaintance of Wesley's apologized:

> I should have wrote to you before myself, but my feelings on the occasion would not permit me to revert to any circumstances respecting her departure, till a gracious Providence had in some measure reconciled me to the afflictive dispensation. I endeavour now to look up to Him with submission, and I bless His name that I find Him my helper.[79]

Another letter, from a bereaved father, announced, "You can weep with those that weep. But I am too much affected to detain you with ceremony. *My children are dead.*" Over three pages, the father struggled with the meaning of his children's death:

> People say "they are taken away from the evil to come." And it is true they are exempt from human miseries. But can we suppose they lose nothing by an early death? They are dismissed the field before the contest begin; can they share a victor's crown?[80]

Dismissing the comforting words of friends, the father concluded that his children's death was a punishment for his own sin.[81] Faced with the prospect of her only child's death, a Methodist widow wrote, "I trust I do *now* give him back to God, my feelings almost seem to unchristianize me."[82]

If, as Methodists feared, feelings could "unchristianize" a believer, grief over the death of a loved one must be continually monitored. Fourteen years after Jacky's death, Wesley wrote a hymn in which he explored his grief again.

1. Solemn, memorable day
That snatch'd my darling son away!
Calm I welcome thy return,
Which summons me again to mourn,
After a sad length of years
To pour again my selfish tears,
To bleed with undiminish'd smart,
And feel the recent wound of heart.

2. Time may gently bring relief,
Assuage or cure a common grief:
I no end of sorrow see,
Till harbour'd in eternity:
Then, my God, and not before,
My penal woes shall all be o'er,
And gloomy sorrow flee away
At the first dawn of endless day.

3. Now, accepting my distress,
I suffer out my evil days;
Softly towards my tomb I tread,
Myself lamenting, not the dead,
Till my life in death appears,
And Jesus, banishing my fears,
Cheers by the beauties of His face,
O'erwhelms me with the glorious blaze.[83]

This hymn presents the suffering of grief as a lifelong burden. It is not triumphantly overcome, like the suffering of persecution, but endured. In emphasizing that his tears were "selfish," and that he was lamenting not his son but himself, Wesley was again marking the limits of acceptable suffering. While he might mourn his own loss, he must not feel sorry for his son, who was happy in heaven. Wesley's only hope was that he too would eventually join his son and be delivered from his suffering.

Again, this hymn presents a somewhat different response to suffering from that depicted in the hymns on pain, persecution and childbirth. In those hymns, resignation is presented as a triumph over suffering, in which the suffering itself almost disappears. Here, by contrast, Wesley described himself as feeling his pain to the full: his resignation came in "accepting" the "distress" of his loss as an ongoing consequence of life as a sinful person in a sinful world. In this hymn the sanctifying value of suffering is not emphasized, there is only a sad resignation to sorrow in this life, and a hope for the end of suffering in the next. Suffering is mastered, not through a triumphant "rising above" the pain, but through an acceptance of its reality within the narrative of life.

While this hymn was written as a response to Wesley's own situation, it also acted as a model for others. That Wesley saw the experience of long-term grieving as legitimate for the Christian is also made clear in a hymn written for the mother of Thomas Waller, a young Methodist man who died in 1781. This hymn, entitled "The Mother's," acts as a model for the experience of bereavement (see Hymn 4). From the outset, it is deeply concerned with the emotional experience of grief, beginning with a plea to be allowed to remember and to mourn:

1. Still let me his remembrance bless,
Still on his dearest image dwell,
Indulge my sorrow's soft excess,
And weep o'er one I loved so well!
Flow fast, and never cease to flow,
Those streams of unforbidden tears,
Till He who shares His creature's woe,
The Comforter in death appears.

That the desire to remember and to weep is framed as a plea suggests that such a desire may be inappropriate. This is reinforced by the use of words such as "indulge" and "excess" to describe the experience of sorrow. But the strength of the desire to weep is overwhelming, and the mother urges her tears to continue flowing unchecked. Tears are "unforbidden," and God is sympathetic to the sufferings of humanity.

This strong expression of grief, accompanied by a certain ambivalence about the value of such emotions, continues in the second verse. Grief forces itself forward again, as again the mother's memory of her son overwhelms her with emotion: "In anguish exquisite I feel,/ I feel the' unutterable loss!" Verse three then provides something of a shift in perspective. The mother's grief is, she reminds herself, for her own loss, not for her son's. If verse one began with the memory of the dead son – an image from the past – verse three replaces this with a new image, this time of the present. Her son is "Safe in the arms of his Beloved/ He looks with pity from the skies." This new image of her son in safety and joy is explicitly given the power to transform the mother's emotions. In verse three, she claims, "His happiness my grief suspends"; in verse four this image or "sense" of his happiness "lulls" her "sorrowing soul to rest." Transformed by the knowledge of her son's salvation, the mother is able to express the resignation of verse five. As in Wesley's anniversary hymn, this verse suggests that mourning will continue for the rest of her life. The "storms of grief" may cease, but her sorrow clearly continues. Again, the hymn ends with an image of the future, of triumphant reunion with her son in the presence of God.

> 5. Not without hope henceforth I mourn;
> (Since Thou, my God, wouldst have it so;)
> He never shall to me return,
> But I ere long to him shall go;
> Thou wilt cut short my mourning days,
> Thou wilt my longing soul prepare,
> To see with him Thy heavenly face,
> And grasp my son triumphant there.

In its vivid depiction of the "storms of grief," this hymn – and others like it – encouraged a space within Methodist culture for the legitimate expression of intense and ongoing grief that might not otherwise have existed. In an early sermon, preached at the funeral of a young man, John Wesley conceded that grief might have some small value in the short term. He warned strongly, however, against the "unprofitable and, by consequence, the sinful nature, of profusely sorrowing for the dead."[84] Famously, in a letter to his sister after the death of all of her children, John wrote:

> I believe the death of your children is a great instance of the goodness of God towards you. You have often mentioned to me how much of your time they take up. Now that time is restored to you and you have nothing to do but serve our Lord till… you are sanctified.[85]

This letter was fairly typical of John's response to grief. Many years later he rebuked a Methodist friend for "inordinate affection" when the friend described his grief over a child's death.[86]

Resignation in the face of bereavement has, of course, been promoted by many devout Christians throughout history.[87] John was, however, particularly strict in his dismissal of the validity or value of lingering grief. If Charles had been similarly inclined to strictness early in life, experience seems to have tempered his views. His letters communicate a strong recognition of the suffering that bereavement brought. In January 1786, he wrote to a friend whose wife had just died:

> Alas, my brother! Are you called to Ezekiel's trial? Son of man, behold I take away from thee the desire of thine eyes with a stroke! A stroke of mere justice, your sorrowful heart tells you: but you shall shortly confess it a stroke of pure mercy! At first you are stunned with it, overwhelmed and confounded.... To feel your loss most sensibly is not a sin; nor even to faint under it as it seems for the present. JESUS WEPT – and allows, and pities all your tears – and will give you patience, till He comes and wipes away all tears from our eyes.[88]

While Charles here conformed to his theological conviction that bereavement must be met with resignation, he legitimized feeling "your loss most sensibly." By offering a model for the expression of grief, his hymns provided a means by which Methodists could sanctify the affliction of grief.

Smallpox, pain, persecution, execution, childbirth, bereavement – Wesley's hymns encouraged Methodists to find in each of these experiences rich meanings, identified by placing experiences of suffering within the narrative of spiritual growth that was so central to early Methodist culture. Within this narrative, suffering could be accepted with resignation because of the assurance that it would ultimately lead to the joy of eternal life. Wesley's hymns acted as tools by which Methodists could assist themselves and others to internalize this assurance when confronted with different experiences of suffering. The hymns represent this process as potentially difficult but always ultimately possible, with God's help.

Early Methodist writings reveal individuals struggling to reflect these ideals, at times succeeding triumphantly, at other times falling short. These writings and Wesley's hymns, however, both depict the process of responding to suffering as one in which the individual was actively involved in shaping his or her own reactions. This analysis suggests that suffering involved "a kind of agency" for early Methodists. The hymns were one tool by which Methodists disciplined themselves within the normative narrative of conversion and sanctification. So far, I have considered the ways in which the hymns focused Methodist energies on personal sanctification in the context of the experience of suffering. The following chapter will examine the ways these energies might be focused outwards, toward the suffering of others.

[Hymn 1]
For One in Pain (Hymn I)

1. Pain, my old companion pain,
Seldom parted from my side,
Welcome to thy seat again,
Here, if God permits, abide:
Pledge of sure-approaching ease,
Haste to stop my wretched breath,
Rugged messenger of peace,
Joyful harbinger of death.

2. Foe to nature as thou art,
I embrace thee as my friend:
Thou shalt bid my griefs depart,
Bring me to my journey's end:
Yes, I joyfully decay,
Homeward through thy help I haste;
Thou hast shook the house of clay;
Surely it will fall at last.

3. Kind remembrancer, to thee
Many a cheerful thought I owe:
Witness of mortality,
Wise through thee my end I know;
Warn'd by every pain I feel
Of my dissolution near;
Pleased the lessening hours I tell:
Quickly shall the last be here.

4. Sacred, salutory ill,
Thee though foolish man miscall,
Mingled by my Father's skill;
Sweet as honey is the gall:
Who beneath thy pressure groan,
Chief of ills who reckon thee,
Sin, alas! they ne'er have known:
Sin is perfect misery.

5. Free from sin I soon shall live,
Free from sin while here below,
Only thou may'st still survive,
Till the joys of heaven I know,
Of my starry crown possess'd;
All thy office then is o'er.
When I gain the glorious rest,
Pain and suffering are no more.[89]

[Hymn 2]

For a Woman near the Time of her Travail

1. To whom should I for succour fly,
While danger, pain, and death are nigh,
And nature's fears return?
Jesus, my only sure relief,
I tell to Thee my secret grief,
And in Thy bosom mourn.

2. I fear, lest in my trying hour
The strength of pain should quite o'erpower
My soul's infirmity,
Lest, when my sorrows most prevail,
My patience and my faith should fail,
And leave me void of Thee.

3. Even now I faint o'erwhelmed with dread,
I tremble at my greatest need
Lest Thou shouldst hide Thy face,
Afflict me more than I can bear,
And then withhold the grace of prayer.
The power to sue for grace.

4. Yet though I am sometimes afraid,
On Thee my feeble mind is stay'd,
My trust is in the Lord,
I hold Thee with a trembling hand,
And borne above myself I stand,
Supported by Thy word.

5. In God my Saviour I confide,
Whose truth and love are on my side;
If now for help I pray,
Thou in the depths of my distress
Wilt send a word of heavenly grace,
And save me through that day.

6. Thou wilt, I humbly trust, impart
The sense of pardon to my heart,
The witness of Thy love:
Thy love shall all my griefs control,
Thy love shall calm my fluttering soul,
And hide my life above.

7. Arm'd with Thy love and patient mind,
I come, to Thy bless'd will resign'd,
For all events prepared,
Soon as I know my pardon seal'd,
Assured that Jesus is my shield,
And infinite reward.[90]

[Hymn 3]
On the Death of a Child.

1. Dead! dead! the child I loved so well!
Transported to the world above!
I need no more my heart conceal:
I never dared indulge my love:
But may I not indulge my grief,
And seek in tears a sad relief?

2. Mine earthly happiness is fled,
His mother's joy, his father's hope:
O had I died in *Isaac*'s stead!
He *should* have lived, my age's prop,
He should have closed his father's eyes,
And follow'd me to paradise.

3. But hath not Heaven, who first bestow'd,
A right to take His gifts away?
I bow me to the sovereign God,
Who snatch'd him from the evil day!
Yet nature *will* repeat the moan,
And fondly cry, "My son, my son!"

4. Turn from him, turn, officious thought!
Officious thought presents again
The thousand little acts he wrought,
Which wound my heart with soothing pain:
His looks, his winning gestures rise,
His waving hands, and laughing eyes!

5. Those waving hands no more shall move,
Those laughing eyes shall smile no more:
He cannot now engage our love
With sweet insinuating power,
Our weak unguarded hearts ensnare,
And rival his Creator there.

6. From us, as we from him, secure,
Caught to his heavenly Father's breast,
He waits, till we the bliss ensure,
From all these stormy sorrows rest,
And see him with our angel stand,
To waft, and welcome us to land.[91]

[Hymn 4]
Part II. The Mother's.

1. Still let me his remembrance bless,
Still on his dearest image dwell,
Indulge my sorrow's soft excess,
And weep o'er one I loved so well!
Flow fast, and never cease to flow,
Those streams of unforbidden tears,
Till He who shares His creature's woe,
The Comforter in death appears.

2. He knows the texture of my heart,
Remembers that I am but dust,
So loath, alas, with that to part
Which nature loves and prizes most!
Partner of all my good and ill,
My friend, my bosom friend, he was,
In anguish exquisite I feel,
I feel the' unutterable loss!

3. Yet for myself, not him, I grieve,
By Mercy's sudden stroke removed,
Beyond the reach of pain to live,
Safe in the arms of his Beloved:
He looks with pity from the skies,
His happiness my grief suspends,
Crown'd with the life that never dies,
Possess'd of joy that never ends.

4. Contemplating his bless'd estate,
I hasten to my endless home,
And lighter feel the' afflictive weight
Which sinks my flesh into the tomb:
The sense of his transcendent bliss
With comfort soothes this aching breast,
Commands these storms of grief to cease,
And lulls my sorrowing soul to rest.

5. Not without hope henceforth I mourn;
(Since Thou, my God, wouldst have it so;)
He never shall to me return,
But I ere long to him shall go;
Thou wilt cut short my mourning days,
Thou wilt my longing soul prepare,
To see with him Thy heavenly face,
And grasp my son triumphant there.[92]

Notes

1. 4 Dec. 1753. *CWJ* 2: 99.

2. 6 Dec. 1753. *CWJ* 2: 100. Sally Wesley contracted the so-called "confluent" smallpox, which was fatal in about 75% of cases. J. R. Smith, *The Speckled Monster: Smallpox in England, 1670–1970, with particular reference to Essex* (Chelmsford: Essex Records Office, 1987), 179–82.

3. *Hymns for the Use of Families* (1767): "Thanksgiving After Recovery from the Small-Pox" and "Another." *PW* 7: 93–95.

4. *Hymns for the Use of Families* (1767): "Thanksgiving After Recovery from the Small-pox." *PW* 7: 94–95.

5. Raymond A. Anselment, *The Realms of Apollo: Literature and Healing in Seventeenth-Century England* (Newark: University of Delaware Press, 1995), 197, 200, 202. See also David Shuttleton, "A Culture of Disfigurement: Imagining Smallpox in the Long Eighteenth Century," in *Framing and Imagining Disease in Cultural History*, ed. George Sebastian Rousseau, Miranda Gill, David Haycock, and Malte Herwig (Basingstoke, Hampshire: Palgrave Macmillan, 2003), 73–74.

6. For a brief introduction to the development of English ideas about sickness and judgment, see Anselment, *Realms of Apollo*, 23–30.

7. Shuttleton, "A Culture of Disfigurement," 73.

8. Shuttleton, "A Culture of Disfigurement," 73.

9. Shuttleton, "A Culture of Disfigurement," 73.

10. See both Anselment, *Realms of Apollo*, 192–211; Shuttleton, "A Culture of Disfigurement," 68–80.

11. Shuttleton, "A Culture of Disfigurement," 76–80.

12. Telford, *The Life of the Rev. Charles Wesley, M.A.*, 197.

13. *SHSPHS* (1762): "Micah 6: 9." *PW* 10: 98. Emphasis in original.

14. John Wesley, "On Divine Providence." Outler, ed., *Sermons II*, vol. 2, *BEW*, 540.

15. Wesley, "On Divine Providence," 542.

16. Wesley, "On Divine Providence," 543.

17. See David Harley, "The Theology of Affliction and the Experience of Sickness in the Godly Family, 1650–1714: The Henrys and Newcomes," in *Religio Medici: Medicine and Religion in Seventeenth-Century England*, ed. Ole Peter Grell and Andrew Cunningham (Aldershot: Scolar Press, 1996), 276.

18. J. W. Haas Jr. "John Wesley's Vision of Science in the Service of Christ," *Perspectives on Science and Christian Faith* 47 (1995): 240.

19. Wesley, "On Divine Providence," 546.

20. Sermon 21: Luke 10: 42. Newport, ed., *Sermons*, 366.

21. See journal entries for 19 Feb. 1750, *CWJ* 2: 68; 19 Feb. 1744, *CWJ* 2: 352; 14 Mar. 1744, *CWJ* 2: 357; 19 July1754, *CWJ* 2: 102; 10 Oct. 1748, *CWJ* 2: 40; 7 May 1741, *CWJ* 1: 274; 18 Mar. 1736, *CWJ* 1: 4; 10 Feb. 1748, *CWJ* 2: 4.

22. *Hymns for the Nation* (1782): "Thanksgiving for the Success of the Gospel in America." *PW* 8: 304–5.

23. The theme of God's providential work through national affliction appears in *Hymns for Times of Trouble and Persecution* (1745), *PW* 4: 1–25; *Hymns Occasioned by the Earthquake* (1750), *PW* 6: 15–35; *Hymns for the Nation* (1782), *PW* 8: 283–355. This understanding was not unique to Wesley, but can be seen as part of the theological context within which evangelical reformers developed their emphasis on ridding the nation of sin. For a discussion of this emphasis in evangelical reform movements, see David W. Bebbington, *Evangelicalism in Modern Britain: A History from the 1730s to the 1980s*

(London: Unwin Hyman, 1989), 132–35; Boyd Hilton, *The Age of Atonement: The Influence of Evangelicalism on Social and Economic Thought, 1785–1865* (Oxford: Clarendon Press, 1988), 209–11.

24. Sermon 21: Luke 10: 42 in Newport, ed., *Sermons*, 366.

25. Elizabeth Marriot to Charles Wesley, nd. DDWES.

26. Mary Guy to Charles Wesley, 14 Jan. 1786. EMV 69.

27. Rachel Hawthorne to Charles Wesley, nd. EMV 84.

28. John Henderson to Charles Wesley, nd. EMV 79.

29. Ann Davis to Charles Wesley, 25 April 1766. EMV 47. Quoted in Phyllis Mack, "Does Gender Matter? Suffering and Salvation in Eighteenth-century Methodism," *Bulletin of the John Rylands University Library of Manchester* 85, nos. 2 and 3 (2003): 169.

30. Mary Purnell to John Wesley, 20 June 1740. Colman Collection.

31. Mack discusses the "agency" involved in suffering in "Does Gender Matter," 174–75.

32. For a discussion of John Wesley's exhortations regarding health care, see Deborah Madden, "Medicine and Moral Reform: The Place of Practical Piety in John Wesley's Art of Physic," *Church History* 73, no. 4 (2004): 741–58.

33. For a good summary of historic Christian attitudes to medicine, see Roy Porter, "Religion and Medicine," in *Companion Encyclopedia of the History of Medicine*, ed. W. F. Bynum and Roy Porter (London: Routledge, 1993), 2: 1449–67.

34. Wesley, *Primitive Physic*, iv.

35. *HSP* (1749): "The Physician's Hymn." *PW* 5: 392–93.

36. Taverner Wallis to Charles Wesley, 27 Nov. 1741. EMV, MARC.

37. See Hempton, *Methodism*, 67; Henry D. Rack, "Evangelical Endings: Death-Beds in Evangelical Biography," *Bulletin of the John Rylands University Library of Manchester* 74, no. 1 (1992): 48.

38. Mack, "Religious Dissenters in Enlightenment England," 8.

39. Mack, "Religious Dissenters in Enlightenment England," 16.

40. Mack, "Religious Dissenters in Enlightenment England," 8.

41. For example, 29 Aug. 1739, *CWJ* 1: 161; 28 Sept. 1739, *CWJ* 1: 182; 22 Sept. 1740, *CWJ* 1: 249; 18 Nov. 1740, *CWJ* 1: 58–61. An extended description of violent opposition to Methodists at Wednesbury is recorded from 2–7 Feb. 1744, *CWJ* 1: 345–48. For a good summary and analysis of animosity toward Methodists, see Paul Langford, *A Polite and Commercial People*, 264–70.

42. 25 Oct. 1743, *CWJ* 1: 340.

43. For examples of hymn-singing in times of persecution, see 18 Nov. 1740, *CWJ* 1: 261; 25 May 1743, *CWJ* 1: 309; 19 July 1744, *CWJ* 1: 370.

44. *HTTP* (1745): "Hymns in Times of Persecution, Hymn V." *PW* 4: 34–35.

45. *HTTP* (1745): "Hymns in Time of Persecution, Hymns I–XIV." *PW* 4: 27–47.

46. *HTTP* (1745): "Hymns in Time of Persecution, Hymns I–XIV." *PW* 4: 27–47.

47. *HTTP* (1745): "Hymns in Time of Persecution, Hymn XII." *PW* 4: 43.

48. John Fletcher, "On the Spiritual Manifestation of the Son of God," *The Arminian Magazine* 16 (June 1793), 318. Quoted in Susan Juster, "Mystical Pregnancy and Holy Bleeding: Visionary Experience in Early Modern Britain and America," *The William and Mary Quarterly* 57, no. 2 (2000): 269.

49. *HSP* (1749): "For the Brethren at the Devizes, Hymn III." *PW* 5: 253.

50. See 12–19 July 1738, *CWJ* 1: 120–24; 11–12 Sept. 1741, *CWJ* 1: 298–99; 22 Feb.–1 Mar. 1748, *CWJ* 2: 6–9; 20–21 Aug. 1753, *CWJ* 2: 94–95.

51. *PCM* (1785): "Hymn IV." *PW* 8: 341–42. In a note on the MS of this series, Wesley wrote, "These prayers were answered. Thursday, April 28th, 1785, on nineteen malefactors, who all died penitent. 'Not unto me, O Lord; not unto me!'"

52. Wesley explicitly identifies execution as an experience of "suffering," which gives support to my contention that he understands suffering as pain that threatens to overwhelm. While the hanging itself might not involve much physical pain, the overall experience of fear, suspense, humiliation and pain could be identified as suffering. For an example of an execution where the repentant condemned men sang hymns repeatedly, see an anonymous "Account of Executions," [nd]. EMV 141.

53. *PCM* (1785): "Hymns 1–13." *PW* 8: 339–50. See also *HSP* (1749): "For Condemned Malefactors." *PW* 4: 460–61 and a number of unpublished hymns for malefactors, *UP* 3: 317–21.

54. Henry D. Rack discusses Methodist attitudes to last-minute conversions in "Evangelical Endings," 47–49.

55. Walsh, "'Methodism' and the Origins of English-Speaking Evangelicalism," 31.

56. See Luke 23: 39–43.

57. *PCM* (1785). "Hymn II." *PW* 8: 340.

58. For a more extensive analysis of the cultural significance of Wesley's hymns for "condemned malefactors," see Joanna Cruickshank, "Singing at the Scaffold: Charles Wesley's Hymns for Condemned Malefactors," *Proceedings of the Wesley Historical Society* 56, no. 3 (October 2007): 129–45.

59. McGowen, "The Body and Punishment," 679.

60. Joshua Fitzsimmonds, *Free and Candid Disquisitions on the Nature and Execution of the Laws of England* (London, 1751), 179, quoted in McGowen, "The Body and Punishment," 662.

61. McGowen, "The Body and Punishment," 679.

62. McGowen, "The Body and Punishment," 675–78.

63. See V. A. C. Gattrell, *The Hanging Tree: Execution and the English People, 1770–1868* (Oxford: Oxford University Press, 1994), 376–82 and Linebaugh, *The London Hanged*, 213–18.

64. McGowen, "The Body and Punishment," 665–66.

65. *PCM* (1785): "Hymn X." *PW* 8: 346.

66. This interpretation is supported by Richard R. Follett's work on evangelicals and penal reform. He demonstrates that the evangelical emphasis on the individual value of human beings gave rise to widespread support for penal reform among evangelicals. See Richard R. Follett, *Evangelicalism, Penal Theory and the Politics of Criminal Law Reform in England, 1808–30* (Basingstoke, Hampshire: Palgrave, 2001), 86.

67. While Wesley wrote hymns for women in childbirth, widows and bereaved mothers, he also wrote hymns for male friends who were sick and for bereaved fathers.

68. Mack, "Does Gender Matter," 163.

69. This criticism by the Victorian hymn-writer Josiah Conder is quoted in Davie, *The Eighteenth-Century Hymn in England*, 64.

70. *Hymns for the Use of Families* (1767) contains more than twenty hymns for women before, during and after childbirth.

71. Charles Wesley to Sally Wesley, 29 Apr. [nd]. DDCW 5/87.

72. *HUF*: "For a Woman in Travail." *PW* 7: 65–66.

73. "Life of Sarah Ryan," 23. MA 24. F/T. Quoted in Mack, "Religious Dissenters," 13.

74. Susanna Designe to John Wesley, 31 Dec. 1741. Colman Collection.

75. "A Short Account of the Death of Daniel Galvin Late of Dublin" to Charles Wesley, 14 Sept. 1748. EMV 62.

76. *Funeral Hymns* (1759): "On the Death of a Child, Part VI." *PW* 6: 259.

77. *HSP* (1749): "On the Death of a Child." *PW* 5: 81–82. There are three more verses in the same style and tone.

78. Sally Wesley to Charles Wesley, 6 July 1768. DDWES 1/50.

79. Unknown author to Charles Wesley, 27 Nov. 1782. DDWES 2/87.

80. John Collinson to Charles Wesley, 11 Sept. 1772. DDWES 1/114.

81. Collinson quoted Ezekiel 18: 2: "The father has eaten sour grapes, and the children's teeth are set on edge."

82. Diaries Collection M, Diary of Mrs. Alexander Mather, 1800–1812, quoted in Mack, "Does Gender Matter," 173.

83. *Hymns and Poems* (unpublished): "Written January 7th, 1768." *PW* 8: 409–10.

84. John Wesley, "On Mourning for the Dead," *BEW* 2: 238.

85. John Wesley to Martha Hall, 1742. Quoted in Rack, *Reasonable Enthusiast*, 542–43.

86. Rack, *Reasonable Enthusiast*, 543.

87. Rack, *Reasonable Enthusiast*, 543.

88. Charles Wesley to Samuel Bradburn, 31 January 1786. DDCW 1/76. For a similarly sympathetic letter of condolence, see Charles Wesley to William Marriot, 22 Sept. 1785. DDCW 7/116. For the death of Ezekiel's wife, see Ezekiel 24: 16.

89. *HSP* (1749): "For One in Pain, Hymn I." *PW* 5: 67–68.

90. *Hymns for the Use of Families* (1767): "For a Woman near the Time of her Travail." *PW* 7: 54–55.

91. *Funeral Hymns* (1759): "On the Death of a Child, Part I." *PW* 6: 252–53.

92. *Funeral Hymns* (unpublished): "The Mother's, Part II." *PW* 6: 347–48.

Chapter Six

Suffering and the Sympathetic Community

In a letter to Sally Gwynne, written in 1747, Charles Wesley declared:

> Those strong expressions of sin and misery which you repeated came from my heart and not my happy brother's. I am peculiarly called to weep with you that weep: and those who suffer most I find as near me as my own soul.[1]

Charles's portrayal of himself in these terms, as he implied, contrasts with contemporary descriptions of his brother John. In 1750, the Methodist layman William Briggs wrote to John, criticizing him for certain spiritual failings: "You have the knowledge of all experience; but not the experience of all you know." As evidence of John's lack of deep spiritual experience, Briggs pointed to:

> the want of sympathy in your discourses and conversations. Those who attend to an inward work more than to an outward, pass through many weighty and grievous conflicts... When do you feelingly and with tears address yourself unto such?[2]

These two descriptions may be used to illuminate the differences between the characters of Charles and John. They contribute to a fairly common portrayal of the two brothers as profoundly different: John as stable, cheerful, unsympathetic; Charles as melancholic, erratic, sensitive to the suffering of others.[3] A closer reading of these descriptions is equally revealing, however, of certain assumptions about the qualities of the ideal Christian. In particular, both letters reveal assumptions about the quality of sympathy, the ability to "weep with you that weep" or to respond "feelingly and with tears" to those who suffer. Both writers assume that such sympathy is a spiritual quality: in Charles's letter it is a "calling"; in Briggs's letter it is essential evidence of the work of the Spirit.

Many of the hymns of Charles Wesley, like these letters, focused on responses to the suffering of others as centrally important to Christian character and virtue. This emphasis is particularly significant in light of the importance given to individual salvation and individual experience in early Methodist culture. Did this emphasis on the individual detract from the formation of community, or could it form the basis of meaningful connections between people? The concept of sympathy provides a key to understanding both Wesley's construction of responses to the suffering of others, and the cultural and theological contexts that shaped this construction.

Sympathy

We have already noted the significance of sympathy within eighteenth-century English culture, in relation to the perceived power of the sight of suffering. The "culture of sensibility" valued both the ability to feel deeply ("sensibility") and the ability to feel deeply for others ("sympathy"). Perhaps the most extensive philosophical exploration of the idea and value of sympathy is found in Adam Smith's *The Theory of Moral Sentiments*. Smith argued that however selfish people might be, they all possessed certain qualities that made them concerned with the needs and happiness of others.

> Of this kind is pity or compassion, the emotion which we feel for the misery of others, when we either see it, or are made to conceive it in a very lively manner. That we often derive sorrow from the sorrow of others, is a matter of fact too obvious to require any instances to prove it; for this sentiment, like all the other original passions of human nature, is by no means confined to the virtuous and the humane, though they may feel it with the most exquisite sensibility. The greatest ruffian, the most hardened violator of the laws of society, is not altogether without it.[4]

For Smith, such empathetic pity for the sufferings of another was one example of sympathy, which he defined broadly as "fellow feeling with any passion whatsoever."[5]

The ability to sympathize with another's experiences was, in Smith's philosophy, a potential "moral sense" and could thus form the foundation for the moral society. Smith's conviction that people shared a common propensity to sympathize with each other's sufferings, and that virtue was reflected in a more "exquisite" or heightened sensibility, can be seen throughout eighteenth-century England. Smith was not the only philosopher to suggest that sympathy could be the basis of a new morality – he was deeply influenced by David Hume, who had earlier affirmed the value of sympathy for society in his *Treatise of Human Nature* (1740). Prior to Hume, the essentially sympathetic nature of human beings had been suggested by Latitudinarian divines of the late seventeenth and early eighteenth centuries.[6]

These philosophical developments echoed ideas within contemporary medical treatises, which explored the "sympathetic" relationship between organs. Markman Ellis points out that during the eighteenth century, the key terms related to the "culture of sensibility" – terms such as "sentiment," "sympathy" and "delicacy" – can also be found throughout "accounts of nerve function, models of the nervous system, accounts of the "circulation" of the blood and theories of the physiological organization of the body as a whole."[7] As will be seen, these portrayals of the body in "sympathetic" terms had significance for understandings of society, which was often conceptualized as a body.[8]

The "culture of sensibility" was perhaps most clearly demonstrated in literary fiction. Novelists such as Samuel Richardson, and later Henry Mackenzie and Laurence Sterne, portrayed heroes and heroines who were men and women of intense feeling.[9] These novels relied on emotive language and heart-rending stories to move the reader to sympathy with these intense characters. Janet Todd describes this "sentimental literature" as "exemplary of emotion, teaching its consumers to produce a response equivalent to the one presented in its episodes."[10] Sentimental literature constructed the ideal person as feeling deeply and sympathizing readily, even involuntarily, with those who suffered. These ideals were explicitly proffered to the reader as models for their own character and responses. In such novels, intense emotion was expressed in an entire "sentimental rhetoric of the body" that included weeping, groaning, blushing, sighing, fainting and an inability to speak.[11] In depicting male heroes in this manner, such literature constructed the ideal man in terms that were conventionally feminine.[12]

Outside the world of fiction, moral reformers used similar literary techniques to portray the suffering of slaves or prisoners or factory workers to attract supporters to their causes. Reformers gave detailed descriptions of physical and emotional suffering to evoke sympathy among readers that would cause them to respond. An example of this kind of writing from within Methodism is found in John Wesley's 1774 essay "Thoughts upon Slavery," which addressed English slave traders:

> Are you a man? Then you should have a human heart. But have you indeed? What is your heart made of? Is there no such principle as compassion there? Do you never feel another's pain? Have you no sympathy, no sense of human woe, no pity for the miserable? When you saw the flowing eyes, the heaving breasts, or the bleeding sides and tortured limbs of your fellow-creatures, was you a stone, or a brute?[13]

As Brycchan Carey has pointed out, the language and style of address that John uses here are typical of contemporary sentimental writing.[14] While these questions are "seemingly addressed to a slave trader and a man of no sensibility... this is an ironic strategy, and the true implied reader is a man of feeling, a man who is shocked by the slave owner's brute insensibility."[15] John's essay was one of the very first uses of sentimental rhetoric in the service of the abolitionist cause.[16]

John's powerful evocation of sympathy in this essay suggests (in spite of criticisms of John as unsympathetic) a relationship between the "culture of sensibility" and the culture of early Methodism. The exact nature of this relationship is, however, complex and contested. As has been noted, the style of Wesley's hymns, with their emphasis on emotional responsiveness, mirrored aspects of the literature of sensibility. Wesley's vivid depictions of the suffering of Christ relied on the sympathetic identification of the viewer for their power. More broadly, Methodists used the language of sensibility in preaching salvation and encouraging reform. For example, in a sermon on the woman taken in adultery, Charles employed many of the techniques of sentimental literature. Calling upon his listeners to consider the woman, he questioned them:

> What says your holiness to an adulteress, a notorious, open sinner? Is pity the first emotion you feel at the sight of her, and do your eyes gush out with water, because she hath not kept God's law? Do you see yourself in her?... Are you thus affected towards her, thus full of pity, sorrow and love, and duly humbled under a sense of your own like sinfulness? Or do you not find the contrary tempers?[17]

Charles argued that the ability to respond to the adulteress with sympathy was the distinguishing characteristic of true holiness. While he elsewhere included many other evidences of holiness, the emphasis here on tearful pity at the sight of the sinner is striking.

In its emphasis on emotional experience, early Methodist culture displayed many of the characteristics of the contemporary culture. There were, however, underlying philosophical tensions between the suggestion that sympathy provided human beings with a natural moral sense and the evangelical claim that all people were inherently sinful and required conversion and transformation. Furthermore, both Methodists and others had to grapple with the question of how sympathy related to moral and charitable action. The Evangelical reformer Hannah More defended sensibility in her early writings, but later condemned its excesses. Sensibility could reduce suffering to an aesthetic experience, and "a feeling heart could justify inaction and excuse error."[18] Christian duty was, More argued, a more reliable motivation for charity. An awareness of this broader "culture of sensibility," and its complicated relationship to Methodism, illuminates the way responses to the suffering of others are constructed within Charles Wesley's hymns.

The Sympathetic Christian

A valuable but neglected source for considering Wesley's portrayal of individual Christians is the group of hymns that Wesley described as "funeral hymns."[19] While some of these were written for use on the death of any believer, many of them eulogize individual Christians, providing lengthy descriptions of the exemplary lives and deaths of the deceased. Many of these individual hymns were not published during Wesley's lifetime, but it seems very likely that they were sung at the funeral of the individual and circulated among family and friends of the deceased. While they include specific details of the lives and experiences of these individuals, they also repeatedly emphasize certain key virtues as characterizing the deceased individuals they commemorate. Those who read and sang the hymns were encouraged to appreciate and develop these characteristics.

These individual funeral hymns are thus a useful indication of how Wesley wanted to construct the ideal Christian.

For the purposes of this analysis, it is significant that Wesley often described in these hymns the ways in which the deceased individual responded to those who suffered. A typical example is found in a hymn entitled "On the Death of Mrs. Mary Naylor, March 21, 1757 (Part III)."

> 1. Mercy, that heaven-descending guest,
> Resided in her gentle breast,
> And full possession kept;
> While listening to the orphan's moan,
> And echoing back the widow's groan,
> She wept with them that wept.
>
> 2. Affliction, poverty, disease,
> Drew out her soul in soft distress
> The wretched to relieve:
> In all the works of love employ'd,
> Her sympathising soul enjoy'd
> The blessedness to give.
>
> 3. Her Saviour in His members seen,
> A stranger she received Him in,
> An hungry Jesus fed,
> Tended her sick imprison'd Lord,
> And flew in all His wants to' afford
> Her ministerial aid.
>
> 4. A nursing mother to the poor,
> For them she husbanded her store,
> Her life, her all bestow'd:
> For them she labour'd day and night,
> In doing good her whole delight,
> In copying after God.
>
> 5. But did she then herself conceal
> From her own flesh? or kindly feel
> Their every want and woe?
> *'Tis Corban this,* she never said,
> But dealt alike her sacred bread
> To feed both friend and foe.[20]

Wesley identified Naylor as possessing (or rather, being possessed by) the quality of mercy. The practical aspect of this virtue – the exercise of charity – is a standard Christian virtue. Wesley's description of Naylor's charitable acts echoes traditional formulations of charity as the service of Christ in the poor.[21] He also, however, emphasized Naylor's sympathetic response to the suffering: "She wept with those who wept." Exposure to the suffering of others "Drew out her soul in soft distress/ The wretched to relieve." The imagery of her soul being "drawn out" implies the almost involuntary reaction of emotion to the sight of suffering that characterized eighteenth-century descriptions of sympathy.[22] In the final verse, Wesley emphasized that her response to the suffering of her own family was similarly sympathetic, as she "kindly" felt "Their every want and woe."

Sympathy is depicted here as closely connected to Christian virtue. It is an aspect of mercy, "that heaven-descending guest," and it is described in specifically biblical terms, as a matter of weeping with those who weep. This portrayal of Naylor also echoes eighteenth-century formulations of the person of "feeling" or "sensibility." Her "gentle breast" and "soft distress," her empathetic response to the "moan" and "groan" of the suffering orphan and widow and her willingness to "kindly feel" the "woe" of her family are all reminiscent of the characters described in the literature of sensibility.

Comparable portrayals of individuals as deeply sympathetic can be found throughout the funeral hymns.[23] Significantly, Wesley portrayed men and women in very similar terms.[24] For example, Wesley writes of Mr. Thomas Lewis:

> 6. His heart, as tender as sincere,
> Melted for every sufferer,
> And bled for the distress'd.
> (Where'er he heard the grieved complain.)
> And pity for the sons of pain
> Resided in his breast.[25]

Like Naylor, Lewis is portrayed in these verses as deeply sympathetic, and his sympathy is described in physical (though metaphorical) terms. His heart was "tender;" it "melted" and "bled" for those who suffered; pity "[r]esided in his breast."

In eulogizing deceased believers in these terms, Wesley constructed the ideal Methodist as one who feels deeply and sympathizes readily. The public singing or private reading of these hymns encouraged early Methodist readers or singers to adopt a similar ideal for themselves and others. Clearly, Wesley's construction of the ideal Methodist echoes broader affirmations of the value of sympathy, particularly as expressed in literary depictions of the "man of feeling." That Wesley depicted men as well as women in these terms supports the contention that Methodism was part of a broader cultural movement that attempted a reformation of manners among English men, a reformation that aimed to replace aggression and violence with tenderness and sympathy.[26]

Wesley portrayed sympathy in thoroughly contemporary terms:

> 1. As in the watery glass
> Face corresponds to face,
> The heart of man to man
> In pleasure and in pain,
> With strictest sympathy agrees,
> And feels the same infirmities.[27]

The idea of sympathy as a correspondence between human hearts "[i]n pleasure and in pain" fits closely with existing understandings of sympathy. Like Smith,

Wesley here implied that sympathy is an attribute common to all human beings rather than a virtue particular to some. Such parallels between the hymns and the broader culture are significant, but they may also be misleading. Wesley's hymns emphasize sympathy within a particular theological framework and for particular spiritual purposes. Without attention to this framework and these purposes, the distinctive nature of Wesley's understanding of sympathy will be missed.

As the funeral hymn for Mary Naylor demonstrates, Wesley emphasized sympathy in the context of a traditional Christian motivation for charity. Sympathy toward the suffering is portrayed in this hymn as one aspect of serving Jesus in the poor.[28] In other funeral hymns, human sympathy is also portrayed as a quality that appropriately imitates the sympathy of Jesus, as in the funeral hymn for Mrs. Mary Horton:

> 1. Say, ye companions of her youth,
> With what sincerity and truth,
> How free from fear or shame,
> Christ and His members she confess'd,
> And through a blameless life express'd
> The tempers of the Lamb.
>
> 2. How did she put His bowels on,
> And answer every plaintive groan
> Of poverty and pain!
> In sad variety of grief
> The wretched sought from her relief,
> Nor ever sought in vain.[29]

The first way in which Horton "express'd/ The tempers of the Lamb" was to sympathize like Jesus, to "put His bowels on" in responding compassionately to the needy. The phrase "bowels of Christ" is here, as elsewhere, used to signify Jesus' emotions, in particular his sympathy and pity. This hymn thus makes clear Wesley's conviction that Christian charity should involve an emotional, sympathetic response to suffering as well as practical action. More significantly, in portraying sympathy as a quality by which the believer imitates Jesus, this hymn points to Wesley's broader representation of Jesus as a deeply sympathetic person.

The Sympathetic Christ

The significance given to sympathy in depictions of Jesus can be seen in a lengthy early hymn entitled "Written in Stress of Temptation" (see Hymn 1). While it does not contain the word "sympathy," a close reading demonstrates that the narrative focuses throughout on sympathetic responses, drawing its readers or singers into a dramatic experience of temptation and salvation.[30] The first six verses of this hymn introduce the narrator as a man overwhelmed by long temptation but continuing to cry out to God. In verses one and two, he describes his plight in biblical phrases that recall the psalmists and the prophets, thus investing his own suffering with profound theological meaning.[31]

1. I am the man who long have known
The fierceness of temptation's rage!
And still to God for help I groan:
When shall my groans His help engage?

2. Out of the deep on Jesus I call,
In bitterness of spirit cry;
Broken upon that Stone I fall,
I fall, – the chief of sinners I.

The narrator describes his emotional pain at length and in detail – his "groans," his "bitterness of spirit," his "sad complaint," the "load of sin" he carries, "the blackness of despair" he feels. His inner struggle against temptation is compared to the struggle of the Gadarene demoniac, possessed by a legion of demons.[32]

If the early verses of the hymn describe the suffering of the narrator, verse seven shifts to a direct and desperate appeal to Jesus. The narrator appeals to the compassion of Christ toward "guilty man," as demonstrated in his Passion: "Thou wouldest not Thy cup decline,/ Thy vengeance due to guilty man." As verse eight makes clear, Christ's own sufferings make him able to empathize with human pain.

8. My sufferings all to Thee are known,
Tempted at every point like me:
Regard my griefs, regard Thine own:
Jesu! remember *Calvary!*

In appealing to this empathetic connection, the narrator makes use of biblical precedent. The writer to the Hebrews affirmed: "we have not an high priest which cannot be touched with the feeling of our infirmities; but was in all points tempted like as we are, yet without sin."[33] Christ's experience of temptation means that the narrator can present his own sufferings as Christ's own: "Regard my griefs, regard Thine own." To prompt Christ's memory with regard to his suffering on Calvary, the narrator launches into a vivid description of those sufferings.

Verses nine to twelve contain a string of emotive references to the Passion.[34] Christ's "agony," his "strong and bitter cries and tears," his "mortal groan," his body "nail'd" to "the tree" – each is urgently brought to his attention. The purpose of this description is clearly to produce a powerful emotional response. In verse ten, for example, Christ is confronted with a series of almost hysterical questions: "For whom didst Thou the cross endure?/ Who nail'd Thy body to the tree?/ Did not Thy death my life procure?" The response that the narrator desires from Christ is not verbal, but emotional: "O, let Thy bowels answer me!" Here Christ's own experience of suffering is posited as the basis by which he is able to feel the sufferings of the narrator: "Canst Thou forget Thy days of flesh?/ Canst Thou *my* miseries not feel?"

The emotive descriptions of these first twelve verses are ostensibly designed to evoke a sympathetic response from Christ: both the narrator's suffering and Christ's own suffering are described to this end. While addressed to Jesus, however, this description also clearly functions to encourage the reader or singer to feel deeply that Jesus is sympathetic to his or her plight. In this way the hymn encourages precisely the emotional sense of Christ's sympathy for which it prays. Verse twelve marks the climax to this emotional crescendo, as Jesus' capacity to sympathize is identified as essential to his nature: "Thy tender heart – it bleeds afresh!/ It bleeds! – *and Thou art Jesus still!*" For Jesus to fail to be sympathetic, these lines imply, would be for him to no longer be himself. It is on the basis of this sympathetic response that Christ is moved to act, transforming the heart of the narrator and thus relieving him from temptation. This transformation is perceived through the emotions: "I feel, I feel Thee now the same!" Because of this perceived transformation, the hymn ends on a note of confident rejoicing.

The portrayal of Christ in "Written in Stress of Temptation" is striking, but not unusual. Similar depictions of Christ as sympathetic fellow-sufferer appear throughout Wesley's hymns.[35] They emphasize pity or compassion as integral to Christ's character and the basis on which he can be appealed to for help. Here the concepts of love and sympathy are almost entirely interchangeable:

1. When shall my grief and pain
Thy kind compassion move?
Thou know'st I languish still to' attain
The happiness of love:
If Thou my suit deny,
Out of Thy presence cast,
Excluded from Thy love, I die,
I die unsaved at last.

2. How shall I plead with Thee,
Saviour of sinful men?
Let Thy own dying love for me
Thy pitying heart constrain:
The universal load,
The cross Thou didst endure
With all the vengeful wrath of God,
To make my pardon sure.[36]

As in the previous hymn, Christ's pity is here seen as central: he is constrained by his "pitying heart" to help the distressed penitent. Once again, the memory of the cross is evoked to move Christ to act. His sacrificial death on the cross is that which most clearly demonstrates his compassionate nature. Reminding him of the sacrifice he made is both a prompt to him identifying with the suffering of the believer and a way of urging him to be true to his nature. Again, the goal of this hymn is the transformation of the narrator, who "languish[es] still to'attain/ The happiness of love." Hymns such as this one repeatedly linked the suffering of Christ, which was elsewhere given such emotional power, to the sympathy of Christ.

In portrayals such as these, Jesus has much in common with the "man of feeling."[37] Like him, Jesus is emotionally responsive to the troubles of others. Like the "man of feeling," too, Jesus expresses this response through physical displays. This can be seen in the references in the hymns to Jesus' tears: Wesley interpreted the famous verse "Jesus wept" as evidence of Jesus' inherently sympathetic nature:

> 1. Jesus weeps, our tears to see!
> Feels the soft infirmity;
> Feels, whene'er a friend we mourn,
> From our bleeding bosom torn;
> Let Him still in spirit groan,
> Make our every grief His own,
> Till we all triumphant rise,
> Call'd to meet Him in the skies.
>
> 2. Jesus weeps for sinners blind,
> Mourns the death of all mankind;
> Blesses us with sacred showers,
> Sheds His tears to hallow ours:
> Weeps to make our case His own,
> For our guilty joys to' atone,
> Wipes at last the mourner's eyes,
> Sorrow's source for ever dries.[38]

In its context, this verse refers to Jesus' response at the death of Lazarus. Historically, Jesus' tears in this account have been interpreted in a myriad of ways. In early modern English sermons on this passage, Christ's tears were understood as demonstrating, variously, grief at Lazarus' death, grief at human doubt, grief at the sin of the world and compassion for Mary and Martha.[39] In this hymn, though Jesus' tears are ascribed multiple meanings, they are primarily a sign of his sympathy for human beings. Jesus weeps in response to human tears. This portrayal is typical of Wesley's treatment of Jesus' tears, which he repeatedly interpreted as evidence of Jesus' pity or sympathy.[40]

This portrayal of Christ clearly resonates with eighteenth-century ideas about sympathy and sensibility. In assuming that because Christ loves, he sympathizes – and that these concepts are almost interchangeable – Wesley was reflecting the assumptions of the "culture of sensibility." Again, however, Wesley's understanding of Christ's ability to sympathize was connected to broader theological themes in the hymns. In particular, Wesley drew direct and indirect connections between his Arminian theology and the sympathy of Jesus. In the hymn above, for example, the lines "Jesus weeps for sinners blind,/ Mourns the death of *all* mankind" clearly contain an attack on limited atonement. This connection is made explicit in one of the anti-Calvinist "Hymns on God's Everlasting Love," published in 1741.

8. Did not His word the fiends expel,
The lepers cleanse, and raise the dead?
Did He not all their sickness heal,
And satisfy their every need?
Did He reject His helpless clay,
Or send them sorrowful away?

9. Nay, but His bowels yearn'd to see
The people hungry, scatter'd, faint;
Nay, but He utter'd over thee
Jerusalem, a true complaint;
Jerusalem, who shedd'st His blood,
That, with His tears, for thee hath flow'd.

10. How oft for thy hard-heartedness
Did Jesus in his Spirit groan!
The things belonging to thy peace,
Hadst thou, O bloody city, known,
Thee, turning in thy gracious day,
He never would have cast away.

11. He wept, because thou *wouldst* not see
The grace which sure salvation brings:
How oft would He have gather'd thee,
And cherish'd underneath His wings;
But thou *wouldst not* – unhappy thou!
And justly art thou harden'd now.[41]

Here Christ's sympathy and compassion toward all those he encountered on earth – his "tears," his "groan," the yearning of his "bowels" – are taken as evidence of his willingness to save anyone who repents. It is this conviction that also underlies the pleading of such hymns as "Written in the Stress of Temptation," which seek to appeal to that sympathetic nature.

The implication that the divine nature is inherently sympathetic is significant in terms of broader theological developments during the late eighteenth and nineteenth centuries. David Bebbington has described the growing evangelical emphasis on the Fatherhood of God during the nineteenth century, an emphasis which meant that ideas of the "paternal pity" of God gained ascendancy over ideas of God's just wrath against sin.[42] While Wesley's hymns emphasized the "vengeful wrath" of God the Father, Jesus was portrayed throughout as compassionate and sympathetic. This emphasis on sympathy as a divine quality seems to prefigure later evangelical portrayals of God as a sympathetic father. In doing so, it points to a tension inherent to evangelical theology, which would only increase over time.

Wesley's hymns portrayed God both as sovereign over suffering (in this life and the next) and, in Christ, as a person of ultimate sympathy. In the hymns, these portrayals act as a source of comfort for the believer, who is able to call out to God who is both sovereign and sympathetic. In later evangelicalism, however, these two doctrines would be seen to conflict: how could a sympathetic

God cause or even allow people to suffer? The growing urgency of this question in nineteenth-century England, particularly as expressed in a rejection of traditional doctrines of hell, has been attested to by a number of historians.[43] Wesley's hymns suggest that the potential for this tension existed within Methodism (and so within evangelicalism more broadly) from its beginnings.

The Sympathetic Body

Jesus' sympathy is also closely connected in the hymns to his relationship with believers. Specifically, Wesley develops the biblical idea of "the body of Christ" as a basis for shared sympathy. Several biblical passages describe the church as the body of Christ – and individual Christians as "members" of this body. A detailed exploration of this concept is found in 1 Corinthians 12: 12, 14, 26:

> For as the body is one, and hath many members, and all the members of that one body, being many, are one body: so also is Christ... And whether one member suffer, all the members suffer with it; or one member be honoured, all the members rejoice with it.

Other biblical passages explore the concept of the church as Christ's body, though elsewhere the connection between shared membership of this body and shared suffering is not emphasized.[44] In Wesley's hymns, however, this connection is repeatedly stressed. Christ's sympathy is seen to derive at least in part from his role as "Head" of the body:

> 1. The members here and Head above,
> United in the Spirit of love
> One mystic body make.
> And Jesus, once a Man of woe
> The sufferings of His saints below
> Doth still in heaven partake.[45]

And, similarly:

> Jesus on the celestial hill
> Doth for his people care,
> Doth suffer in His members still,
> And all our sorrows bear:
> If crush'd on earth the foot complain,
> Feeling the injury
> The Head above cries out in pain,
> "Thou persecutest Me."[46]

The idea of spiritual unity or "membership" of Jesus' "body" seems in Wesley's thought to be almost inseparable from the experience of suffering. Jesus continues to partake in the suffering of believers: he "suffers in His members still."

The boundary between sympathy and unity is here blurred: Jesus actually enters into the pain of his suffering people.[47]

Not surprisingly, this emphasis upon the sympathetic nature of the body of Jesus has great significance for Wesley's portrayal of the Christian community. Sympathy was a central element in his ideal Christian community, as can be seen in a lengthy poem on "The Communion of Saints":

> 4. Sweetly now we all agree,
> Touch'd with softest sympathy,
> Kindly for each other care:
> Every member feels its share:
> Wounded by the grief of one,
> All the suffering members groan;
> Honour'd if one member is,
> All partake the common bliss.[48]

Here "membership" of the body is the basis of a profound sympathetic connection. In this portrayal, the members' responses to each other's pains are given far more prominence than their responses to each other's pleasures. This emphasis on the sympathetic nature of the Christian community is repeated in many of Wesley's hymns.[49]

In emphasizing the sympathetic connections between members of a metaphorical body, Wesley reflected a broader shift within eighteenth-century discourses surrounding both the body and society. Again, this is demonstrated in contemporary debates over the value and nature of corporal and capital punishment. As has been noted, these debates reflected two opposing and incompatible views of society. Defenders of public execution repeatedly compared society to the human body, a metaphor that served to emphasize both the interdependence and the distinctly demarcated roles of individuals within society.[50] For the reformers who opposed public execution, however, individuals were connected not by duty and hierarchy, but by "interest and feeling," which grew out of the shared experience of being an embodied individual. Society, for these reformers, "constituted a community founded on sympathy."[51] In this framing, society was understood less in terms of a metaphorical body politic, and more in terms of the physical bodies of individuals.

In Wesley's portrayal of the Christian community, the metaphor of the body is used repeatedly, but not to reinforce traditional notions of a hierarchical society. The biblical passages that describe the church as a "body" use the metaphor to emphasize both the diversity of roles in the church and the sympathetic connections that should bind its members together. It is therefore significant that Wesley, in his use of this metaphor, emphasized sympathy over diversity and interdependence. Other than recognizing the role of Christ as "Head" of the body, Wesley rarely mentioned the diversity of functions within the body.[52] As has been mentioned, eighteenth-century medical theories did interpret bodily functions in terms of "sympathetic" connections. Wesley's construction of the community of believers made use of this understanding: believers share in one another's pleasures and, particularly, pains.

Rising out of the spiritual reality of shared membership of Jesus' body, sympathy is portrayed as a quality that distinguishes the Christian community from all others. A hymn on "Desiring to Love" expresses this clearly (see Hymn 2), presenting Jesus as deeply sympathetic toward the suffering believer.

> 1. O Saviour, cast a pitying eye,
> A sinner at Thy feet I lie,
> And will not hence depart,
> Till Thou regard my ceaseless moan;
> O speak, and take away the stone,
> The unbelieving heart:

This divine sympathy is mirrored by the sympathy of the supplicant's fellow-believers. They enter into the suffering of the one desiring to love: they "bear" "my cross," they "feel my care." Again, the "body of Christ" is the theological context for these sympathetic responses: "The suffering members sympathise,/ And grieve my griefs, and sigh my sighs." Their sympathy is contrasted starkly with the attitude of those in "the world," who "admire" the supplicant's grief but cannot sympathize with it. Sympathy unites, but it also divides.

This hymn also identifies, however, the potential limits of sympathy in Wesley's understanding.

> 7. But all in vain for me they grieve,
> Their sufferings cannot mine relieve,
> Or mitigate my pain:
> No answer to their prayers they see,
> And prevalent with God for me
> They seem to pray in vain.
>
> 8. Thou then, O God, Thine hand lay to,
> And let me all the means look through,
> And trust to Thee alone,
> To Thee alone for all things trust,
> And say to Thee, who sav'st the lost,
> Thine only will be done.

As verse seven makes clear, the sympathy of the supplicant's fellow-believers is ultimately "all in vain." Their empathetic sufferings, and even the supplications that they are moved to pray, are ineffective. Only God can minister to the deep need of the narrator. The repeated use of the words "alone" and "only" in the final verse emphasizes that it is God's intervention that ultimately makes a difference, not the "means" of the community's sympathy and prayers. This final verse implies a warning that the sympathy of other Christians, while comforting, must not be relied upon for that which only God can provide. This hymn and others caution that the sympathetic fellowship offered by the Christian community could become idolatrous.[53]

While for Wesley the shared membership of Jesus' body meant that Christians would be particularly sympathetic toward each other, the hymns also emphasize the importance of sympathy toward all who suffer. In a "Hymn for the National Fast," written in 1782, in the context of war with America, Wesley wrote:

3. With every sufferer,
We drop the generous tear,
(Whom Thy tendering Spirit leads,)
Pity no distinction knows,
Love for all the wounded bleeds,
Love embraces friends and foes.[54]

The "tendering Spirit" leads Christians into an all-embracing sympathy. Even those American rebels whom Wesley identified as "foes" are included in this embrace. Sympathy here becomes not only the means by which believers express love for each other, but also the means by which believers relate to those across boundaries of belief, race and nationality.[55]

Charity and Sympathy

Throughout Wesley's hymns, then, the ideal Christian is constructed as deeply sympathetic. This construction relies on the assumption that the loving person, led by "the tendering Spirit," is able to experience in some way the sufferings of another person – regardless of status, religion or race. In Wesley's hymns, as in the philosophical discussions of Adam Smith and others, this ability provided an obvious motivation for charitable action. Especially in the funeral hymns, but elsewhere as well, sympathy leads to charity. One example is the funeral hymn for Mrs. Mary Naylor: "In all the works of love employ'd/ Her sympathising soul enjoy'd/ The blessedness to give."[56] The relationship between sympathy and Christian charity was not, however, straightforward. Traditional Christian exhortations to charity were concerned as much with duty as with sympathy.[57] As evangelical critics such as Hannah More argued, sympathy could be indulged at the expense of practical assistance.[58]

Wesley's hymns reflected both older and newer visions of charity. In one of Wesley's few hymns on the subject of charity, entitled "In the Work [of Charity]," a complicated picture emerges (see Hymn 3). From the beginning, this hymn presents charity as an experience with multiple meanings.

1. I come, O God, to do Thy will,
With Jesus in my view,
A pattern of His servants still,
My Pattern I pursue.

2. My loving labour I repeat,
Obedient to His word,
And wash His dear disciples' feet,
And wait upon my Lord.

The opening lines suggest that the narrator of this hymn is to approach the work of charity obediently, but also "with Jesus in my view." What it means to have "Jesus in my view" is more complicated than may first appear. The straightforward meaning of this phrase is presented in this first verse: Jesus offers a pattern for charity, and so is kept "in view" as a model during the work of charity. But verse two complicates matters: here the act of charity is not simply a matter of copying Jesus, who washed his disciples' feet, but also of serving him directly – "And wait upon my Lord." As the hymn goes on to make clear, Jesus is also "in my view" during the work of charity in that it provides a context in which he may be encountered. In the work of charity, the hymn claims, Jesus can be seen.

Verses three to nine reinforce this idea by expanding on a number of Biblical phrases and passages. The most significant is from Matthew 25: 35–46, where Jesus assures his disciples that those who care for the needy – by visiting them in prison, by feeding them or giving them water – are in fact serving him. This is a traditional biblical basis for exhortations to charity, and verses four to eight give an extended description of charity in these terms. In doing so, they shift the reader's attention back and forth between the person of the poor man and the person of Jesus. This shift in focus is indicated by the use of capitals: Wesley denotes Christ as "Him," while "him" refers to an ordinary human being. In verse four, then, the body shivering and exposed, the hands helplessly held out, these are really the body and hands of Christ. What other possible response to this sight, the hymn asks, than for us to give of our wealth to help the one who has spiritually clothed us? The first nine verses seem to act as an emotional crescendo, in which the narrator's response to the suffering – pity at their plight – is carefully entwined with his or her response to Christ – guilt and gratitude to the one who saves.

If these first verses are a crescendo, verses ten to twelve represent both a climax and a sudden shift in focus.

10. My needy Jesus I descry,
And in this object meet,
Sick, and in pain I see Him lie,
And gasping at my feet.

11. Paleness His dying face o'erspreads,
His griefs I more than see,
My heart at Jesu's suffering bleeds
With softest sympathy.

12. I fill my Lord's afflictions up,
His welcome burden bear,
And gladly drink His bitter cup,
And all His sorrows share.

The emotional intensity increases, as the reader is confronted with a description of much more extreme suffering. The adjectives pile up: "sick," "in pain," gasping," "pale," "dying," "suffering." The appropriate response to this sight, as the hymn makes explicit, is the "softest sympathy." This evocation of intense sympathy marks a sudden shift in the direction of the hymn as a whole as, in verse twelve, the narrator begins suffering. He or she is described as though on the cross with Jesus, sharing his "afflictions," bearing his "burden," drinking the "bitter cup" of God's judgment, sharing all of Christ's "sorrows."

This moment of intense identification with Christ is brief, but it changes the direction of the hymn significantly. The poor person, who has never been a very distinct identity within this hymn, disappears almost entirely. He or she is mentioned as "this object" in verse ten, and then is gone from view. In addition, the narrator is suddenly seeing more clearly. There are a couple of references to sight in the first half of the hymn, but from now on they become repetitive. In verse ten, "I descry," "I see him lie"; in verse eleven, "I more than see"; in verse thirteen, "I now behold Thy face"; in verse fourteen, "Mine eyes of faith survey"; in verse fifteen, "might it now appear"; in verse sixteen, "and see and serve, as I do now." Through the moment of intense, almost mystical sympathy in verse twelve, the spiritual eyes of the narrator have been opened. Jesus' suffering body – his "visage marr'd with tears and blood," his body "torn with the whips, and nails and spears" – is on view to the believer. To see this, verses thirteen and fourteen suggest, is to understand the theological significance of Jesus' suffering: that he "suffered in my place," as "a bleeding Victim" of God's justice. For Wesley, this understanding was central to spiritual change. The hymn therefore ends with the evangelistic concern that the whole world should see and understand Jesus' suffering, and serve him in the act of charity.

This hymn is concerned with both sympathy and charity, but the relationship between the two is not straightforward. While sympathy is given enormous power and significance in this hymn, it does not operate as a direct motivation for charity. Without denying the possibilities of sympathy, the explicit motivations given for charity in verses one and two are obedience and love of Christ. The basis of charity in the following verses is the traditional Christian rationale of serving Christ in the poor and suffering. The body and emotions of the suffering man himself are somehow distanced from us, the readers or singers of the hymn. Sympathy is powerfully evoked throughout this hymn, but it is primarily evoked in response to the sufferings of Christ. Human suffering is only a dim reflection of the overwhelming suffering of Christ. At no point do we "see" the suffering man himself. Rather, we see Christ in him. Charity in this hymn is firstly a matter of serving and knowing Christ, and only secondly a matter of serving and knowing fellow human beings.

As a model for charity, this hymn provides a powerful incentive for the care of those in need. Such care is given profound spiritual value within the framework of Christian love and obedience. At the same time, the first half of this hymn suggests a certain discomfort at the unmediated sight of human suffering, or at least an ambivalence about the value of such a sight. What is important for Wesley is not that which is physically seen, but that which is spiritually seen, that which the believing person perceives with the "eyes of faith." Such an approach to charity might be useful where what was seen was too repulsive to elicit compassion, but it could also presumably result in the needs and experience of the individual being overlooked.

The portrayals of charity here and in the funeral hymns represent alternative constructions of the place of sympathy in Christian charity. In the funeral hymns, the care of others is often portrayed as proceeding from the sympathetic response of a sanctified heart. Sympathy in this context is a fruit of the spirit, but it is also an appropriate motivation for charity. In this earlier (and more extended) exploration of charity, care of others rests on an older formulation in which charity was an opportunity for service to Christ. This depiction of the poor as "members of Christ" is more strongly found in John Wesley's writings.[59] Overall, the plight of the poor is a more obvious theme in John's writings than in Charles'.[60] In Charles's hymns, the poor are certainly depicted as "members of Christ," but the overall emphasis on sympathy as a motivation for charity suggests that Charles increasingly understood charity in these terms.

As has been noted, the promotion of sympathy as a particular virtue valued within the broader culture of eighteenth-century England, but in Wesley's hymns it is given a particular, Christological interpretation. Jesus is presented as inherently sympathetic, and his sufferings are presented as both source and expression of this sympathy. Believers, individually and as a community, suffer and sympathize in imitation of a suffering and sympathetic Lord. This Christological framework also places limits on sympathy within the hymns. The broader uneasiness within evangelicalism about the power of sympathy is mirrored in Wesley's insistence that human sympathy must not be relied on to provide that spiritual good which only God can provide. Sympathy in the hymns could be humanitarian, but it could never be humanist.

The Sympathetic Methodist

The construction of the ideal Methodist in these terms has real significance for illuminating certain distinctive aspects of early Methodist culture. It is a commonplace that Methodism was concerned with individual experience but, as Hindmarsh has argued, "if the converts in the early Evangelical Revival appear as individualists of a sort, they were also communitarians of a sort."[61] The Methodist conversion narratives he examines reveal that many individuals were drawn to the intense experience of community that early Methodism offered.[62] The writers of these narratives repeatedly mention the value of the fellowship they experienced in the intimate settings of band and society meetings. These meetings provided a context within which those who were seeking salvation or greater holiness could share their experiences, comfort, challenge and pray for one another. Such shared practices were explicitly identified as "means of grace."[63] My analysis has supported Hindmarsh's contention that such practices assisted Methodists in interpreting the events of their lives within meaningful personal narratives.

Like many aspects of early Methodism, this intense community can be seen in part as a response to the particular social and cultural conditions in which eighteenth-century English people lived. Early English Methodism often (though not always) thrived in areas where old ties to squire and parson had been loosened, often because of broader social changes involving population growth and mobility.[64] In this context, Methodism offered an alternative community, based on alternative loyalties. This was clear to contemporary critics of the movement:

> It is really no light evil for a state to have within its bosom so numerous, active and increasing a party, whose whole system tends to cut them off from all common sympathy with their fellow countrymen, and who are separatists, not in religious worship alone, but in all the ordinary observations of life.[65]

For this commentator, the "common sympathy" of the nation was threatened by a community based not on shared national identity but on the perception of a shared experience of conversion and sanctification, pointing to a shared identity as members of Christ's body.[66]

This spiritual experience and identity challenged social distinctions as well as social unity. In preaching justification by faith and the necessity of conversion: "Methodists, Congregationalists and Baptists… propagated a spiritual status system which, while not radical in any political sense, cut across the hierarchical structures of the contemporary society."[67] Evangelical theology claimed that all people had sinful hearts and that all people needed to be justified by faith. Methodists and other Arminian evangelicals went further in saying that all people *could* be justified by faith: there was no inherent distinction between the saved and the unsaved. As expressed in Methodist culture, this theology meant that every individual's life could be mapped along the same basic narrative: whatever their experiences, the underlying meanings of their lives were the same. A person might respond to God or not, but the true story of their life was one of God's continual gracious call to repentance, faith and holiness.

Charles Wesley's emphasis on sympathy grew out of this context and affirms it. In a community gathered around the shared (and often painful) experience of conviction, conversion and the struggle for sanctification in the midst of the pains of daily life, sympathy provided a powerful cohesive force. Its expression affirmed the shared nature of these experiences and so their validity. Wesley's letters are full of his appreciation for the intensity of Methodist fellowship, and his hymns encouraged Methodists to develop the quality of sympathy that contributed to this intensity.[68] Through hymns that depicted Jesus as profoundly sympathetic, Methodists were encouraged to associate divine love with the practice of sympathy. Through funeral hymns that lauded the sympathetic nature of deceased believers, they were provided with exemplars of the sympathetic person of feeling. Through the emphasis on shared membership of Christ's body, they were assured that they could truly sympathize with each other's sufferings because these sufferings were ultimately part of a shared spiritual story and identity. More broadly, through repeatedly singing hymns that emphasized the ultimate commonality of human experience, they were encouraged to believe that just as salvation was offered to all, so all could be sympathized with.

There is evidence to suggest that sympathy did become a significant element in Methodist identity. Consider, for example, the Methodist response to the campaign for the abolition of slavery in the early nineteenth century. Methodists were deeply involved in this campaign, and proved the most committed of all emancipationist groups.[69] The reasons for this involvement are hotly debated and clearly complex: certainly, the English abolition of slavery cannot simply be attributed to Methodist sympathy.[70] Most early English Methodists had, however, never been to the West Indies, or watched slaves being packed into a slave ship for transportation, or seen slaves at work on a plantation. Their knowledge of this suffering came from its literary evocation in the writings of anti-slavery reformers, writings that increasingly conformed to the conventions of the literature of sensibility in seeking to evoke sympathetic responses from "persons of feeling." English Methodists were clearly responsive to these portrayals, and involved in their dissemination.

Thomas Clarkson, perhaps the most influential figure in the English anti-slavery movement, described the role of Methodist ministers in the movement as promoting "a softness of feeling" toward American slaves.[71] Charles Wesley's hymns certainly encouraged Methodists to see "softness of feeling" toward others as a central Christian virtue. The theological connection that Charles drew between an Arminian confidence in the possibility of salvation for all and a sympathetic portrayal of God may also illuminate the comparative responsiveness to abolitionism of Arminian evangelicals over Calvinists.[72]

Paul Langford notes that the late eighteenth-century abolitionist campaign, which appealed primarily to the "sensibility" of the middle class, was unable to effect significant reform. He concludes, "[i]t needed the somewhat harder core of moral earnestness provided by the evangelicals to turn it into a weapon of real weight and effectiveness."[73] The ideal Christian constructed in Wesley's hymns, who was sympathetic in a theological context that emphasized the perils of sinfulness for the nation, the liberty of the individual will and the need for personal activism, seems ideally placed to engage with the abolitionist cause.[74] Of course, if early Methodists did strive to develop and act upon their sensitivity to the suffering of others, there is also evidence to suggest that their sympathy could be selective.[75]

To "weep with you that weep" was, for Charles Wesley, not only a high personal calling, but also a mark of true Christian character and community. In constructing the ideal Methodist as deeply sympathetic, Wesley's hymns resonate powerfully with broader cultural trends in eighteenth-century England. They also encourage the formation of a new, distinctively Methodist identity, one that would aim to follow a sympathetic Lord in weeping "for all mankind." The potential tensions in his portrayal, however – between the judgment and the compassion of God, between the sympathy and the duty of Christians, between the spiritual equality of all people and the temporal distinctions among them, between loyalty to other believers and sympathy for all – are tensions that would be felt within evangelical theology and practice for centuries to come.

[Hymn 1]
Written in Stress of Temptation

1. I am the man who long have known
The fierceness of temptation's rage!
And still to God for help I groan:
When shall my groans His help engage?

2. Out of the deep on Jesus I call,
In bitterness of spirit cry;
Broken upon that Stone I fall,
I fall, – the chief of sinners I.

3. Saviour of me, my sad complaint
Let me into Thy bosom pour;
Beneath my load of sin I faint,
And hell is ready to devour.

4. A devil to myself I am,
Yet cannot 'scape the flesh I tear;
Beast, fiend, and legion is my name,
My lot the blackness of despair.
. . . .

7. My Lord, (I still will call Thee mine,
Till sentenced to eternal pain,)
Thou wouldest not Thy cup decline,
Thy vengeance due to guilty man.

8. My sufferings all to Thee are known,
Tempted at every point like me:
Regard my griefs, regard Thine own:
Jesu! remember *Calvary!*

9. O, call to mind Thy earnest prayers,
Thine agony and sweat of blood,
Thy strong and bitter cries and tears,
Thy mortal groan, "MY GOD! MY GOD!"

10. For whom didst Thou the cross endure?
Who nail'd Thy body to the tree?
Did not Thy death my life procure?
O, let Thy bowels answer me!

11. Art Thou not touch'd with human woe?
Hath pity left the Son of Man?
Dost Thou not all our sorrow know,
And claim a share in all our pain?

12. Canst Thou forget Thy days of flesh?
Canst Thou *my* miseries not feel?

Thy tender heart – it bleeds afresh!
It bleeds! – and Thou art Jesus still!

13. I feel, I feel Thee now the same,
Kindled Thy kind relentings are;
These meltings from Thy bowels came,
Thy Spirit groan'd this inward prayer.

14. Thy prayer is heard, Thy will is done!
Light in Thy light at length I see;
Thou wilt preserve my soul Thine own,
And show forth all Thy power in me.[76]

[Hymn 2]
Desiring to Love

1. O Saviour, cast a pitying eye,
A sinner at Thy feet I lie,
And will not hence depart,
Till Thou regard my ceaseless moan;
O speak, and take away the stone,
The unbelieving heart:

2. Till Thou the mountain load remove,
I groan beneath my want of love;
O hear my bitter cry:
Without Thy love I cannot live,
Give, Jesus, Friend of sinners, give
Me love, or else I die.

3. Dost Thou not all my sufferings know,
Dost Thou not see mine eye o'erflow,
My labouring bosom move?
Why do I all this burden bear?
Need I to Thee the cause declare?
Thou know'st, I cannot love.

4. This is my sin and misery,
I always find Thy love to me,
Seal'd by Thy precious blood;
And yet I make Thee no return,
I only for my baseness mourn,
I cannot love my God.

5. The world admire my mystic grief,
And torture me with vain relief,
And cruel kindness show;
They bid me give my wailings o'er,
And weep and vex myself no more
For One they never knew.

6. My Father's children feel my care,
With kind concern my cross they bear,
And in my sorrows join;
The suffering members sympathise,
And grieve my griefs, and sigh my sighs.
And mix their tears with mine.

7. But all in vain for me they grieve,
Their sufferings cannot mine relieve,
Or mitigate my pain:
No answer to their prayers they see,
And prevalent with God for me
They seem to pray in vain.

8. Thou then, O God, Thine hand lay to,
And let me all the means look through,
And trust to Thee alone,
To Thee alone for all things trust,
And say to Thee, who sav'st the lost,
Thine only will be done.[77]

[Hymn 3]
In the Work [of Charity]

1. I come, O God, to do Thy will,
With Jesus in my view,
A pattern of His servants still,
My Pattern I pursue.

2. My loving labour I repeat,
Obedient to His word,
And wash His dear disciples' feet,
And wait upon my Lord.

3. I have my Saviour always near,
On Him I now attend,
I see Him in His members here,
My Brother, and my Friend.

4. Shivering beneath those rags He stands,
Again exposed, and bare,
And stretches out His helpless hands,
And asks my tender care.

5. And shall I not relief afford,
Put off my costly dress,
Tear it away to clothe my Lord,
Who hides my sinfulness!

6. Drink to a thirsty Christ I give,
An hungry Christ I feed,
The stranger to my house receive.
Who here shall lay his head.

7. Sick and in prison will I find,
And all his sorrows cheer,
Or bring him forth, and doubly kind
Relieve, and tend him here.
…

9. Surely I now my Saviour see,
In this poor worm conceal'd,
Wounded He asks relief of me,
Who all my wounds hath heal'd.

10. My needy Jesus I descry,
And in this object meet,
Sick, and in pain I see Him lie,
And gasping at my feet.

11. Paleness His dying face o'erspreads,
His griefs I more than see,
My heart at Jesu's suffering bleeds
With softest sympathy.

12. I fill my Lord's afflictions up,
His welcome burden bear,
And gladly drink His bitter cup,
And all His sorrows share.

13. Yes, Lord, with joy, and grief, and love
I now behold Thy face,
My God descended from above
To suffer in my place.

14. Thy visage marr'd with tears and blood,
Mine eyes of faith survey,
As when on yonder cross my God
A bleeding Victim lay.

15. Torn with the whips, and nails, and spear
Thy sacred body was;
O might it now to all appear
As hanging on the cross!

16. O that to Thee the world might bow,
And know Thy saving name,
And see, and serve, as I do now,
And love the bleeding Lamb! [78]

Notes

1. Charles Wesley to Sarah Gwynne, 17 Nov. 1747. DDCW 5/3.

2. William Briggs to John Wesley, 5 Apr. 1750. Colman Collection.

3. For one example of such a portrayal, in an introduction to Methodism, see Barrie Tabraham, *The Making of Methodism* (London: Epworth, 1995), 11.

4. Smith, *The Theory of Moral Sentiments*, 9.

5. Smith, *The Theory of Moral Sentiments*, 9.

6. A number of examples are quoted by Halttunen, "Humanitarianism and the Pornography of Pain in Anglo-American Culture," 304–5.

7. Markman Ellis, *The Politics of Sensibility: Race, Gender and Commerce in the Sentimental Novel* (New York: Cambridge University Press, 1996), 18–19.

8. McGowen, "The Body and Punishment in Eighteenth-Century England," 675.

9. For example, Henry Mackenzie, *The Man of Feeling* (London, 1771), Laurence Sterne, *A Sentimental Journey through France and Italy* (London, 1768) and Samuel Richardson, *Pamela: or Virtue Rewarded* (London, 1740). As Langford points out, the "sensibility" of later writers such as Sterne represented a more powerful defense of "the primacy of an individual's feelings" than the work of earlier sentimental novelists like Richardson. Langford, *A Polite and Commercial People: England*, 463–64.

10. Todd, *Sensibility*, 4.

11. Ellis, *The Politics of Sensibility*, 19.

12. For discussions of sensibility and gender, see Barker-Benfield, *The Culture of* Sensibility; Todd, *Sensibility*.

13. John Wesley, "Thoughts upon Slavery," in *Political Writings of John Wesley*, ed. Graham Maddox (Bristol: Thoemmes Press, 1998), 103.

14. Carey, "John Wesley's *Thoughts upon Slavery*," 278–84.

15. Carey, "John Wesley's *Thoughts upon Slavery*," 283–84.

16. Carey, "John Wesley's *Thoughts upon Slavery*," 284.

17. Sermon 10. John 8:1–11. Newport, ed., *Sermons*, 254–55.

18. Todd, *Sensibility*, 64, 137. Hannah More criticized "sentiment" in "On the Danger of Sentimental or Romantic Connexions" (1778).

19. Wesley published two collections of *Funeral Hymns* (1746, 1759) and wrote many more funeral hymns that remained unpublished during his lifetime. See *PW* 6: 188–366.

20. *Funeral Hymns* (1759): "On the Death of Mrs. Mary Naylor. Part III." *PW* 6: 270–71.

21. For traditional views of charity in England, and the way these views changed during the eighteenth century, see Deborah Valenze, "Charity, Custom and Humanity: Changing Attitudes towards the Poor in Eighteenth-Century England," in *Revival and Religion since 1700: Essays for John Walsh*, ed. Jane Garnett and Colin Matthew (London, Rio Grande: Hambledon Press, 1993), 59–78.

22. See Fiering, "Irresistible Compassion," 195–218.

23. Funeral hymns that portray the deceased as sympathetic include *Funeral Hymns* (unpublished): "On the Death of Mr. Thomas Hogg, June 29, 1750." *PW* 6: 290–91; "On the Death of Lady Hotham, June 30, 1756 (Part III)." *PW* 6: 296; "On the Death of Mr. John Matthews, December 28, 1764." *PW* 6: 308–13; "On the Death of Mrs. Hannah Dewal." *PW* 6: 318–23; "On the Death of Mrs. Elizabeth Blackwell, March 27, 1772." *PW* 6: 323–31; "On the Death of Mr. Thomas Waller, In his Thirtieth Year, May 11, 1781." *PW* 6: 345–461; "On the Death of Mr. Ebenezer Blackwell, April 21, 1782." *PW* 6: 353–55.

24. See, for example, *Funeral Hymns* (unpublished): "On the Death of Mr. Thomas Waller, In his Thirtieth Year, May 11, 1781." *PW* 6: 345–46 and "On the Death of Mr. Ebenezer Blackwell, April 21, 1782." *PW* 6: 353–55.

25. *Funeral Hymns* (unpublished): "On the Death of Mr. Thomas Lewis, April, 1782." *PW* 6: 350.

26. Barker-Benfield, *The Culture of Sensibility*, 266–79.

27. *SHSPHS* (1762): "Acts 14: 15." *PW* 12: 290–91. In Acts 14: 15, Paul and Barnabas dissuade the people of Lystra from treating them as gods by saying "We also are men of like passions with you." In the biblical context this has little to do with sympathy.

28. Other hymns that communicate this understanding of charity include *HSP* (1749): "Before Any Work of Charity" and "For One in the Work." *PW* 5: 18–21.

29. *Funeral Hymns* (unpublished): "On the Death of Mrs. Mary Horton, May 4, 1786, Aged Thirty-four (Part III)." *PW* 6: 359–60. There are eight verses in all.

30. I refer to the central figure of this narrative as "the narrator." As the title identifies this figure with Charles himself (and because Charles writes "I am the *man*...") I have used masculine pronouns in referring to him.

31. Lamentations 3: 1, Psalm 130: 1–2, Isaiah 28: 16 (the latter verse is also quoted in 1 Peter 2: 6–8, and Wesley is obviously following this Christological interpretation).

32. Luke 8: 26–39.

33. Hebrews 4: 15.

34. There are a number of sources for this description. The Church of England Litany refers to "Thy agony, Thy bloody sweat." Wesley also seems to be referring to Hebrews 5: 7 – "Who in the days of his flesh, when he had offered up prayers and supplications with strong crying and tears unto him that was able to save him from death, and was heard in that he feared."

35. A small selection of examples from many hymns that portray Jesus in these terms includes *PW* 1: 83–85; *PW* 2: 156–58; *PW* 4: 250; *PW* 5: 231–32; *PW* 9 :34; *PW* 11: 118; *PW* 11: 223; *PW* 12: 104.

36. *Hymns for Love* (nd): "Hymn IX." *PW* 8: 363. There are two more verses.

37. This similarity is noted in Todd, *Sensibility*, 50.

38. *SHSPHS* (1762): "John 9: 35." *PW* 11: 475–76.

39. Marjory E. Lange, *Telling Tears in the English Renaissance* (Leiden: E. J. Brill, 1996), 157–86.

40. See *PW* 1: 330–32, 11: 223, 11: 233, 11: 268–69.

41. *Hymns on God's Everlasting Love* (1741): "Hymn X." *PW* 3: 20–23.

42. Bebbington, *The Dominance of Evangelicalism*, 166–69.

43. Bebbington, *The Dominance of Evangelicalism*, 171. Lucy Bending, *The Representation of Bodily Pain in Late Nineteenth-Century English Culture* (Oxford: Clarendon Press, 2000), 5–27.

44. For example, see Romans 12: 4–5 and Ephesians 4: 15–16.

45. *SHSPHS* (1762): "Acts 9: 4." *PW* 12: 234. There are two more verses.

46. *SHSPHS* (1762): "Zechariah 2; 8." *PW* 10: 112. Zechariah 2: 8: "He that toucheth you toucheth the apple of His eye."

47. In this context, it may be significant that Wesley writes about the church as the body of Jesus, rather than the body of Christ, given that the use of the name "Jesus" emphasizes his embodied nature.

48. *HSP* (1740): "The Communion of Saints, Part IV." *PW* 1: 362.

49. For example, *PW* 1: 298–99, *PW* 2: 164–66, *PW* 3: 173–74, *PW* 4: 473–74, *PW* 5: 78.

50. McGowen, "The Body and Punishment," 679.

51. McGowen, "The Body and Punishment," 675.

52. Diversity within the Christian body is mentioned in *HSP* (1740): "The Communion of Saints, Part IV." *PW* 1: 362.

53. For another example of a cautious approach to sympathy in the hymns, see *HSP* (1740): "Upon Parting with His Friends, Part II." *PW* 1: 245–46.

54. *Hymns for the National Fast* (1782): "Hymn VIII." *PW* 8: 324.

55. Other examples of sympathy for enemies include *PW* 4: 28, *PW* 8: 335.

56. *Funeral Hymns* (1759): "On the Death of Mrs. Mary Naylor, March 21, 1757." *PW* 6: 270.

57. See Valenze, "Charity, Custom and Humanity," 62–63.

58. Todd, *Sensibility*, 137–41.

59. John Walsh, "John Wesley and the Community of Goods," in *Protestant Evangelicalism: Britain, Ireland, Germany and America c.1750–c.1950*, ed. Keith Robbins, *Studies in Church History* (Oxford: Basil Blackwell, 1990), 35.

60. For a comparison of the brothers' attitudes to the poor, see Lloyd, "Charles Wesley: A New Evaluation of his Life and Ministry," 177–79.

61. Hindmarsh, *The Evangelical Conversion Narrative*, 150.

62. Hindmarsh, *The Evangelical Conversion Narrative*, 150–56.

63. Hindmarsh, *The Evangelical Conversion Narrative*. 151.

64. Hempton, *Methodism*, 17–30. See also Walsh, "'Methodism' and the Origins of English-Speaking Evangelicalism," 30–32. For a more sociological analysis of Methodism's "capacity for satisfying the profound associational and communal needs of people experiencing anomie and social insecurity in a period of rapid social change and dislocation," see Alan D Gilbert, *Religion and Society in Industrial England: Church, Chapel and Social Change 1740–1914* (London: Longman, 1976), 87–93.

65. E. T., *Methodism Exposed* (1813), 1. Quoted in van Noppen, *Transforming Words*, 165–66.

66. As Paul Langford points out, the Methodist tendency to form a separate community within established communities was one of the main causes of hostility toward the movement. Langford, *A Polite and Commercial People*, 267.

67. Gilbert, *Religion and Society*, 83.

68. For examples of Charles's description of intense times of fellowship see Charles Wesley to Sarah Gwynne, 5, 6 Feb [1749]. DDCW 5/25; Charles Wesley to Sarah Wesley, 26 Sept. [1757]. DDCW 5/75; Charles Wesley to Sarah Wesley, 8 Sept. [1757]. DDCW 5/104.

69. Hempton and Walsh, "E.P. Thompson and Methodism," 113. For the involvement of Methodists (and other evangelicals) in the anti-slavery campaigns, see Adam Hochschild, *Bury the Chains: Prophets and Rebels in the Fight to Free an Empire's Slaves* (Boston: Houghton Mifflin, 2005), chapters 9, 22.

70. For a discussion of some alternative explanations for Methodist responsiveness to the abolition campaigns, see David Hempton, *The Religion of the People: Methodism and Popular Religion, c.1750–1900* (London: Routledge, 1996), 163–64. Abolitionists noted that they received the greatest response from their hearers when they stressed the sinfulness of the slave trade. See Bebbington, *Evangelicalism in Modern Britain*, 133.

71. Thomas Clarkson, *History of the rise, progress and accomplishment of the abolition of the African slave trade*, 2 vols., vol. 1 (London: Longman, Hurst, Rees and Orme, 1808), 170–171. Quoted in Carey, "John Wesley's *Thoughts upon Slavery*," 276. Carey argues convincingly that Clarkson underestimated the role of the Methodist leadership, but it remains significant that Clarkson chose to describe their role in these particular terms.

72. Hempton, *Methodism*, endnote 15, 234.

73. Langford, *A Polite and Commercial People*, 318.

74. Also, as one contemporary evangelical leader noted, the sympathies of evangelicals were directed toward the "external circumstances of the oppressed and miserable of all lands" through the experience of overseas mission. Richard Watson, quoted in Hempton, *The Religion of the People*, 165.

75. For example, American Methodists, particularly in the South, soon abandoned their strong stance against slavery. Mark A. Noll, *The Rise of Evangelicalism: The Age of Edwards, Whitefield and the Wesleys* (Downers Grove, Ill.: Inter-Varsity Press, 2003), 255.

76. *HSP* (1740): "Written in Stress of Temptation." *PW* 1: 273–76.

77. *HSP* (1749): "Desiring to Love, Hymn III." *PW* 4: 338–39.

78. *HSP* (1749): "In the Work." *PW* 5: 19–21.

Conclusion

Charles Wesley and Early Methodism

Writing to his son in 1838, the Congregationalist hymn-writer Josiah Conder quoted from a hymn of Charles Wesley's, and then explained:

> I did not insert the hymn in our collection, because it is unsuitable for congregational use; and like many other beautiful hymns of almost impassioned devotion, by the same author, it savours too much of the mystic school of piety, which is not the Pauline. There is nothing monastic, feminine, or mawkish, in the fervent devotion of the Apostle, to his Master and Lord... Now the devotion of the Romish mystic, from which that of Wesley and Zinzendorf was borrowed as regards its style, is not of this masculine fibre, of this daylight character.[1]

There are few things upon which an eighteenth-century Methodist, a nineteenth-century Congregationalist and a twentieth-century Marxist could be expected to agree. In making this criticism, however, Conder expressed similar opinions to those articulated by John Wesley, writing forty years earlier, and E. P. Thompson, who would analyze Methodism 125 years later. From very different perspectives, these men concluded that Charles Wesley's hymns were overly "mystic," "feminine," "melancholy" and, in Thompson's more damning judgment, "masochistic."[2] Whatever the theological, literary or psychological merit of these criticisms, the discomfort they express is, I suggest, related to the distinctive aspect of Charles Wesley's hymns that this book has examined: his construction of suffering. Analyzing this construction has illuminated not only the attempts of one eighteenth-century individual to interpret and manage pain, but also the culture of the early English Methodists who read and sang his works.

Wesley's understanding of suffering may be summarized in terms of doctrine, by extracting a systematic theology of suffering from the propositional statements about affliction contained in his hymns. The theology that has emerged from my analysis is not so much systematic as poetic, relying not on a series of logical connections, but rather on a series of parallels and paradoxes. Through the sin of Adam, all humanity is doomed to suffer; through the suffering of Christ, all humanity is offered freedom from sin. Christ demonstrated his perfection through a life of submissive suffering; Christians reach perfection through an imitative life of submissive suffering. In Christ, God is revealed as one who sympathizes with those who suffer; in Christ, the "members" of his body take on his sympathizing character. While none of these propositions are original, together they contribute to a theology that gave great importance to the suffering of Christ and Christians, to a degree unusual within Protestant theology. In particular, in emphasizing the role of suffering in sanctification, Charles developed a theology of perfection that was noticeably different from that presented by his brother John. My analysis thus supports recognition both of the theological diversity within early Methodism, and of Charles Wesley as a theologian in his own right.

As I have argued, however, such an approach to the hymns is only partially adequate. Wesley's hymns were not simply theological statements, but tools for producing and managing experience. They were designed to draw people into the "narrative culture" of Methodism, by engaging their singers or readers in stories of personal transformation that linked to an overarching narrative of conviction, conversion, sanctification and eternal glory. Wesley's hymns thus represent a particular construction of the experience of suffering and its place in the Christian life. Those who read and sang the hymns were encouraged to adopt both a spirituality and a story in which suffering had great importance.

The spirituality that Wesley constructed was centered on the sufferings of Christ. Wesley's depiction of the Passion of Christ communicated a complicated message about suffering: its inevitable presence in the world as God's judgment on sin, as well as its redemptive possibilities in the hands of a loving God. To encounter the suffering Christ was thus to be confronted by the gospel message of God's justice and grace. Such an encounter would be shocking, overwhelming, and ultimately transformative. The hymns repeatedly evoke the sight of the suffering Christ to this end.

This depiction of the sufferings of Jesus and their spiritual meanings contributed to an understanding of the self as naturally "hard-hearted" – both emotionally and spiritually unresponsive to the love and authority of God. Wesley's hymns engaged the reader or singer in a story about this self, a narrative in which suffering was part of the solution to spiritual intransigence. The hymns encouraged believers to expect a life of suffering that paralleled the sufferings of Christ. Such suffering would be agonizing and overwhelming but, as the individual submitted him or herself to the will of God, it would result in the purification and perfection of the self. This perfection of the self would mean becoming, like Christ, soft-hearted and sympathetic toward all who suffer.

The criticisms that John Wesley, Josiah Conder and E. P. Thompson leveled at Charles's hymns are helpful clues to historicizing this construction. In developing a spirituality of the suffering Christ, Charles drew on a long tradition of Passion devotion, which had its roots in the late medieval period. His emphasis on the confronting "sight" of this suffering melded this older tradition with eighteenth-century anxieties about the effect of seeing suffering bodies. While many evangelical hymns (including Conder's own) depicted the sufferings of Christ, few hymn-writers, apart from the Moravians, described these sufferings so repeatedly, so passionately and in so much detail as Charles Wesley. And few evangelical hymns were so insistent that this suffering must be paralleled in intensity by the suffering of Christians. This focus could easily be condemned as "Romish" or "mystical" devotion. It certainly provoked John Wesley's and E. P. Thompson's criticisms of Charles's "melancholy" and "masochistic" depiction of life.

For both Conder and Thompson, Charles's imagery and style was inappropriately "feminine." These claims support my argument linking Wesley's hymns to the broader "culture of sensibility" within eighteenth-century England. The emphasis throughout the hymns on emotional responsiveness, the depiction of Christ and his people as deeply sympathetic, as well as the power given to the sight of others in pain, all reflect a wider cultural shift that gave increasing value to the capacity to feel deeply. As numerous historians have pointed out, this shift constructed the ideal human being in terms that were conventionally feminine. In reflecting this shift, Wesley's hymns can be seen as part of a broader "feminization of piety": their role in this trend deserves further consideration.[3] However, Wesley's depiction of sympathy also included reservations about the place of sympathy in the Christian life, pointing to broader evangelical concerns about the cultural significance of sensibility. By the mid-nineteenth century, when Conder wrote, Victorian evangelicals were expressing strong anxieties about the dangers of "effeminacy."[4] Clearly, the submissive, sensible, suffering voice, which the hymns made normative for believers, heightened these fears.

Moving to the broader questions the preceding chapters have addressed, what does the construction of suffering in the hymns reveal about early English Methodism? As I have argued throughout, the hymns themselves can only give a "top-down" view of Methodism: assuming that they are exactly representative of Methodist experience and conviction ignores the diversity of Methodist culture and the reality of individual agency within the movement. Reading the hymns in the context of the letters and journals of early Methodists has confirmed this view. Methodist men and women interpreted their experiences of suffering in ways that both reflected and diverged from the construction of suffering in the hymns.

The suffering of Christ was, clearly, a central aspect of Methodist spirituality. We have noted many examples of men and women who recorded their transformative encounters with the suffering Jesus, their identification with him in the midst of pain and the love and gratitude they felt toward him for his sacrifice. The hymns gave a formal voice to this devotion, shaping and encouraging its expression without directly threatening Protestant prohibitions against images of the divine. While the particular shape and intensity of Methodist devotion to the crucified Christ may have been distinctive, such devotion is not surprising, given standard definitions of evangelicalism, which include "crucicentrism," a focus on the atoning work of Christ in his death on the cross.[5] The particular construction of responses to Christ's suffering in Wesley's hymns, and its parallels in Methodist culture, demonstrates the importance of exploring crucicentrism as not only a theological characteristic, but a cultural one, expressed in the experience of life, relationships and religious devotion, as well as in formal doctrine.

Wesley's hymns contributed to a crucicentric culture, in which a powerful apprehension of the sufferings of Christ linked into a narrative of individual experience that emphasized the penitential struggle that preceded conversion and the life of imitative suffering that followed it. Not all Methodists found that their experiences conformed to this norm, as demonstrated by the Methodist preacher who was surprised to find that his conversion was not preceded by "horrible fears and terrors."[6] Nonetheless, many men and women did interpret their sufferings within this narrative. The language of "cup," "cross" and "furnace" demonstrates people's desire to understand their sufferings as imitative and sanctifying, while the overarching story of the "cross" leading to the "crown" could give meaning to hardship and encourage perseverance in difficult times.

Constructing individual experience in terms of this narrative could lead to either a passive acceptance of injustice or wholehearted social activism – or sometimes both. Awareness of the construction of suffering in the hymns helps to illuminate the complicated, seemingly contradictory, responses of Methodists to authority. The narrative contained in the hymns was, as E. P. Thompson recognized, inherently political in its emphasis on absolute submission to God through the experience of suffering. But it was neither inherently conservative nor inherently progressive: the "way of the cross" was lived out in complicated relationship with the society and culture of those who embraced it.[7] The experiences of Methodists who committed to living out this story must be interpreted on their own terms if they are to be understood.

Wesley's hymns offered not just a framework for interpreting suffering in general, but a plethora of specific responses to individual experiences of pain and hardship. Where they made use of these hymns, early Methodists were developing an identity that, if not stable or unchanging, related to eighteenth-century culture in distinctive ways. Wesley's hymns offered responses to experiences as diverse as childbirth, execution, grief and smallpox. These hymns put words to experiences that might otherwise have been inexpressible. Without arguing that Wesley's responses were adopted fully by early Methodists, his emphasis on the overarching purposes of Providence, the need for resignation, the value of sympathy, the acceptability of grief and the importance of the individual are all aspects that can be identified in early Methodism, as well as in the evangelicalism of the following centuries. In particular, the repeated emphasis on the value of sympathy has significance for understanding Methodist involvement in social reform.

As I have also noted, however, the normative experience of sanctification constructed in the hymns was unusual in its emphasis on extreme suffering. This emphasis was criticized from within Methodism itself, and does not seem to have been adopted fully by most Methodists. As Methodism became increasingly respectable in its membership, this emphasis probably became even more distasteful. This is certainly suggested by George Osborn's comment, in his edition of Wesley's works, that "every judicious reader" would reject Wesley's insistence on the need for Christians to suffer.[8] Similar constructions of the Christian life would continue to emerge in the "holiness" movements that descended from Methodism but, like Wesley's vision, would not long survive.[9]

This book opened with an account of unimaginable pain, asking how such suffering could be endured, and why experiences such as these mattered so much to early Methodists. I conclude by reflecting on another account of individual suffering. Writing to Charles Wesley in 1766, Mrs. Anne Davis (probably the same Mrs. Davis whose mastectomy had been described to him eight years earlier) declared that she was "oppressed beyond expression with this painful body." She confessed:

> [I]t is a time of sore trial and temptation with me. I see much of my want of faith and every grace of the Spirit and the blessing of a closer union with the Lord Jesus, that I may be enabled through faith in him to tread in his steps and be a thankful partaker of his sufferings without a stammering groan.[10]

At times Mrs. Davis struggled to achieve resignation, but: "hitherto the Lord hath helped me. . . he gives me to hope he will make me more than conqueror at last."

For Mrs. Davis, suffering, and her responses to suffering, mattered. Charles Wesley's hymns help explain why. His hymns were designed both to heighten and alleviate the kind of anxieties that Mrs. Davis experienced, when faced with overwhelming pain of the mind and body. The hymns placed her experience of suffering within an ongoing spiritual drama, where the stakes were eternal. This made suffering an experience of great spiritual concern. The hymns also offered, in their broad construction of suffering and in their depiction of specific instances of affliction, tools by which this suffering could be sanctified. Anne Davis's desire for intimacy with Christ, her understanding of pain as an opportunity to imitate him, her determination to submit to suffering "without a stammering groan" and her hope of victory "at last" all conform to the construction found in Wesley's hymns.

Appropriately, therefore, when Ann Davis died, Charles Wesley wrote her a funeral hymn, which begins:

> 1. Glory to God on high!
> The God whom saints adore
> Hath caught our partner to the sky,
> And sorrow is no more:
> The long, dark hour is past,
> And, lo, to sight restored,
> She gains the dazzling prize at last,
> And sees her smiling Lord.[11]

The final verse is a prayer that when "faith hath pass'd the fire," those singing will join Mrs. Davis "To spend, in praises of our God/ A blest eternity."

The language of the hymn suggests that, in addition to Mrs. Davis's other troubles, she was blind for at least part of her life. Wesley's hymns encouraged early Methodists to believe that blindness, like a "breast being cut out," childbirth, persecution, betrayal and a host of other pains that threatened to overwhelm the believer, were part of the process by which a "closer union with the Lord Jesus" and, ultimately, a "dazzling prize" could be gained. If for some this assurance seemed dangerously mystical, feminine or masochistic, for others it meant the strength to endure suffering, in the hope of being "more than conqueror at last."

Notes

1. Josiah Conder, quoted in Davie, *The Eighteenth-Century Hymn in England*, 64.

2. For John Wesley's and E. P. Thompson's criticisms of Charles's hymns, see Thompson, *The Making of the English Working Class*, 406-11; Ward and Heitzenrater, eds., *Journal and Diaries VII (1787–91)*, vol. 24, *BEW*, 117.

3. Callum G. Brown, *The Death of Christian Britain: Understanding Secularisation, 1800–2000* (London, New York: Routledge, 2001), 58–87. For an alternative argument, see Robert B. Shoemaker, *Gender in English Society, 1650–1850: Men and Women, Separate Spheres?* (London, New York: Longman, 1989), 222–25.

4. Leonore Davidoff and Catherine Hall, *Family Fortunes: Men and Women of the Middle Class, 1780–1850* (Chicago: University of Chicago Press, 1987), 109–14.

5. Bebbington, *Evangelicalism in Modern Britain*, 14–17.

6. George Story's experience is discussed in Chapter Three and found in Stephens, ed., *Lives of the Early Methodist Preachers*, 101.

7. For a superb example of analysis of the relationship between the "way of the cross" and a particular culture, see Schneider, *The Way of the Cross Leads Home*.

8. For Osborn's criticisms, see *PW* 13: 157.

9. For an example, see Bebbington, *Evangelicalism in Modern Britain*, 16.

10. Ann Davis to Charles Wesley, 25 April 1766. EMV 47.

11. *Funeral Hymns* (unpublished): "On the Death of Mrs. Ann Davis, November 5th, 1775." *PW* 6: 338–39.

Bibliography

Manuscripts

Methodist Archives and Research Centre (MARC), John Rylands University Library, Manchester

Charles Wesley Papers (DDCW 1–7).
Early Methodist Volume (EMV).
Fletcher-Tooth Collection (F/T).
Wesley Family Papers (DDWES 1, 2, 4).

Printed Primary Sources

Chilcote, Paul Wesley, ed. *Her Own Story: Autobiographical Portraits of Early Methodist Women.* Nashville: Abingdon, 2001.

Kassler, Michael and Philip Olleson, ed. *Samuel Wesley (1766–1837): A Source Book.* Aldershot: Ashgate, 2001.

Smith, Adam. *The Theory of Moral Sentiments*, edited by D. D. Raphael and A. L. Macfie. London: 1759. Reprinted Oxford: Oxford University Press, 1976.

Tyson, John R., ed. *Charles Wesley: A Reader*. New York: Oxford University Press, 1989.

Wainwright, Arthur W., ed. *Wesley-Langshaw Correspondence: Charles Wesley, His Sons and the Lancaster Organists*. Emory: Scholars Press, 1993.

Wesley, Charles. *The Sermons of Charles Wesley: A Critical Edition with Introduction and Notes*, edited by Kenneth G. C. Newport. Oxford: Oxford University Press, 2001.

———. *The Unpublished Poetry of Charles Wesley*, edited by S. T. Kimbrough and Oliver A. Beckerlegge. 3 vols. Nashville: Kingswood Books, 1988–92.

———. *The Journal of the Rev. Charles Wesley, M.A., Sometime Student of Christ Church, Oxford*, edited by Thomas Jackson. 2 vols. London: John Mason, 1849. Reprinted Grand Rapids, Michigan: Baker Book House, 1980.

Wesley, Charles, and John Wesley. *The Poetical Works of John and Charles Wesley*, edited by George Osborn. 14 vols. London: Wesleyan-Methodist Conference Office, 1868–72.

Wesley, John. *The Bicentennial Edition of the Works of John Wesley*, gen. eds. Frank Baker and Richard P. Heitzenrater. 26 vols. Nashville: Abingdon Press, 1976–.

———. *Political Writings of John Wesley*, edited by Graham Maddox. Bristol: Thoemmes Press, 1998.

Wesley, Susanna. *Susanna Wesley: The Complete Writings*, edited by Charles Wallace. Oxford, New York: Oxford University Press, 1997.

Articles and Monographs

Adey, Lionel. *Class and Idol in the English Hymn*. Vancouver: University of British Columbia Press, 1988.

Amato, Joseph. *Victims and Values: A History and Theory of Suffering*. New York: Greenwood Press, 1990.

Anselment, Raymond A. *The Realms of Apollo: Literature and Healing in Seventeenth-Century England*. Newark: University of Delaware Press, 1995.

Arnold, Richard. *The English Hymn: Studies in a Genre*. New York: Peter Lang, 1995.

Ashworth, John. "The Relationship between Capitalism and Humanitarianism." *The American Historical Review* 92, no. 4 (1987): 813–28.

Baker, Frank. *Charles Wesley's Verse: An Introduction*. Second ed. London: Epworth Press, 1988.

———. "A Poet in Love: The Courtship of Charles Wesley, 1747–1749." *Methodist History* 29, no. 4 (1991): 235–47.

———. *Representative Verse of Charles Wesley*. London: Epworth Press, 1962.

Barker-Benfield, G. J. *The Culture of Sensibility: Sex and Society in Eighteenth-Century Britain*. Chicago: University of Chicago Press, 1992.

Bebbington, David W. *The Dominance of Evangelicalism: The Age of Spurgeon and Moody*. Downers Grove, Ill.: Inter-Varsity Press, 2005.

———. *Evangelicalism in Modern Britain: A History from the 1730s to the 1980s*. London: Unwin Hyman, 1989.

Bending, Lucy. *The Representation of Bodily Pain in Late Nineteenth-Century English Culture*. Oxford: Clarendon Press, 2000.

Bennett, J. A. W. *Poetry of the Passion: Studies in Twelve Centuries of English Verse*. Oxford: Clarendon Press, 1982.

Berger, Teresa. *Theology in Hymns? A Study of the Relationship of Doxology and Theology According to A Collection of Hymns for the People Called Methodists*, translated by Timothy E. Kimbrough. Nashville: Kingswood Books, 1995.

Bett, Henry. *The Hymns of Methodism*. London: Epworth Press, 1945.

Brailsford, Mabel Richmond. *A Tale of Two Brothers: John and Charles Wesley*. London: Rupert Hart-Davies, 1954.

Brantley, Richard E. *Locke, Wesley and the Method of English Romanticism*: Gainesville: University Presses of Florida, 1984.

Brown-Lawson, Albert. *John Wesley and the Anglican Evangelicals of the Eighteenth Century*. Durham: The Pentland Press, 1994.

Carey, Brycchan. "John Wesley's *Thoughts upon Slavery* and the Language of the Heart." *Bulletin of the John Rylands University Library of Manchester* 85, nos. 2 and 3 (2003): 269–84.

Clapper, Gregory S. *John Wesley on Religious Affections: His Views on Experience and Emotion and Their Role in the Christian Life and Theology*. Metuchen, N.J., and London: Scarecrow Press, Inc., 1989.

Cruickshank, Joanna. "'Appear as Crucified for Me': Sight, Suffering and Spiritual Transformation in the Hymns of Charles Wesley." *Journal of Religious History* 30, no. 3 (2006): 311–30.

———. "Singing at the Scaffold: Charles Wesley's Hymns for Condemned Malefactors." *Proceedings of the Wesley Historical Society* 56, no. 3 (October 2007): 129–45.

Dallimore, Arnold A. *A Heart Set Free: The Life of Charles Wesley*. Welwyn: Evangelical Press, 1988.

Davidoff, Leonore, and Catherine Hall. *Family Fortunes: Men and Women of the Middle Class, 1780–1850*. Chicago: University of Chicago Press, 1987.

Davie, Donald. *The Eighteenth-Century Hymn in England*. Cambridge: Cambridge University Press, 1993.

Dreyer, Frederick. "Faith and Experience in the Thought of John Wesley." *The American Historical Review* 88, no. 1 (1983): 12–30.

Duffy, Eamon. *The Stripping of the Altars: Traditional Religion in England, c. 1400–c. 1580*. New Haven, London: Yale University Press, 1992.

Ellis, Markman. *The Politics of Sensibility: Race, Gender and Commerce in the Sentimental Novel*. New York: Cambridge University Press, 1996.

Fiering, Norman S. "Irresistible Compassion: An Aspect of Eighteenth-Century Sympathy and Humanitarianism." *Journal of the History of Ideas* 37, no. 2 (Apr.–June 1976): 195–218.

Flew, Robert Newton. *The Hymns of Charles Wesley: A Study of Their Structure*. London: Epworth Press, 1953.

Follett, Richard R. *Evangelicalism, Penal Theory and the Politics of Criminal Law Reform in England, 1808–30*. Basingstoke, Hampshire: Palgrave, 2001.

Gilbert, Alan D. *Religion and Society in Industrial England: Church, Chapel and Social Change 1740–1914*. London: Longman, 1976.

Gill, Frederick C. *Charles Wesley: The First Methodist*. London: Lutterworth Press, 1964.

Gregory, Jeremy. "Charles Wesley and the Eighteenth Century." Pages 18–39 in *Charles Wesley: Life, Literature and Legacy*, edited by Kenneth Newport and Ted Campbell. Peterborough: Epworth, 2007.

Hadden Hobbs, June. *"I Sing for I Cannot Be Silent": The Feminization of American Hymnody*. Pittsburgh: University of Pittsburgh Press, 1997.

Halttunen, Karen. "Humanitarianism and the Pornography of Pain in Anglo-American Culture." *The American Historical Review* 100, no. 2 (1995): 303–34.

Hammond, Geordan. "Restoring Primitive Christianity: John Wesley and Georgia, 1735–1737." PhD diss., University of Manchester, 2008.

Harley, David. "The Theology of Affliction and the Experience of Sickness in the Godly Family, 1650–1714: The Henrys and Newcomes." Pages 273–92 in *Religio Medici: Medicine and Religion in Seventeenth Century England*, edited by Ole Peter Grell and Andrew Cunningham. Aldershot: Scolar Press, 1996.

Haskell, Thomas L. "Capitalism and the Origins of Humanitarian Sensibility, Part 1." *The American Historical Review* 90, no. 2 (1985): 339–61.

———. "Capitalism and the Origins of Humanitarian Sensibility, Part 2." *The American Historical Review* 90, no. 3 (1985): 547–66.

Hempton, David. *Methodism and Politics in British Society, 1750–1850*. London: Hutchinson, 1984.

———. *Methodism: Empire of the Spirit*. New Haven and London: Yale University Press, 2005.

———. *The Religion of the People: Methodism and Popular Religion, c.1750–1900*. London: Routledge, 1996.

Hempton, David, and John Walsh. "E. P. Thompson and Methodism." Pages 99–122 in *God and Mammon: Protestants, Money, and the Market, 1790–1860*, edited by Mark A. Noll. Oxford: Oxford University Press, 2002.

Hill, A. Wesley. *John Wesley Among the Physicians: A Study of Eighteenth-Century Medicine*. London: Epworth Press, 1958.

Hilton, Boyd. *The Age of Atonement: The Influence of Evangelicalism on Social and Economic Thought, 1785–1865*. Oxford: Clarendon Press, 1988.

Hindmarsh, D. Bruce. *The Evangelical Conversion Narrative: Spiritual Autobiography in Early Modern England*. New York: Oxford University Press, 2005.

———. "'My Chains Fell Off, My Heart Was Free': Early Methodist Conversion Narrative in England." *Church History* 68, no. 4 (1999): 910–29.

Hochschild, Adam. *Bury the Chains: Prophets and Rebels in the Fight to Free an Empire's Slaves*. Boston: Houghton Mifflin, 2005.

Irelan, Rebecca. "A Little Experiment in Practical Divinity: Charles Sanders Peirce and the Women of Early Methodism Socialize the Subject of John Wesley's Doctrine of Sanctification." PhD diss., Graduate Theological Union, 2008.

Jackson, Thomas. *The Life of the Rev. Charles Wesley*. 2 vols. London: Wesleyan Methodist Conference Office, 1841.

Jones, D. M. *Charles Wesley: A Study*. London: Skeffington, 1919.

Juster, Susan. "Mystical Pregnancy and Holy Bleeding: Visionary Experience in Early Modern Britain and America." *The William and Mary Quarterly* 57, no. 2 (2000): 249–88.

Kimbrough, S. T. *Lost in Wonder: Charles Wesley, The Meaning of His Hymns Today*. Nashville: The Upper Room, 1987.

———, ed. *Charles Wesley: Poet and Theologian*. Nashville: Abingdon, 1992.

Lange, Marjory E. *Telling Tears in the English Renaissance*. Leiden: E. J. Brill, 1996.

Langford, Paul. *A Polite and Commercial People: England, 1727–1783*. Oxford: Clarendon Press, 1989.

Linebaugh, Peter. *The London Hanged: Crime and Civil Society in the Eighteenth Century*. London: Penguin, 1991.

Lloyd, Gareth. "Charles Wesley and His Biographers: An Exercise in Methodist Hagiography." *Bulletin of the John Rylands University Library of Manchester* 82, no. 1 (2000): 81–100.

———. "Charles Wesley: A New Evaluation of his Life and Ministry." PhD diss., University of Liverpool, 2002.

———. *Charles Wesley and the Struggle for Methodist Identity*. Oxford: Oxford University Press, 2007.

Lobody, D. H. "'That Language Might Be Given Me': Women's Experience in Early Methodism." In *Perspectives on American Methodism: Interpretive Essays*, edited by E. Richey. Nashville: Abingdon Press, 1993.

MacDonald, A. A., H. N. B. Ridderbos, and R. M. Schlusemann, eds. *The Broken Body: Passion Devotion in Late Medieval Culture*. Groningen: Egbert Forsten, 1998.

Mack, Phyllis. "Does Gender Matter? Suffering and Salvation in Eighteenth-century Methodism." *Bulletin of the John Rylands University Library of Manchester* 85, nos. 2 and 3 (2003): 157–76.

———. "Religious Dissenters in Enlightenment England." *History Workshop Journal* 49 (2000): 1–23.

Madden, Deborah. "Medicine and Moral Reform: The Place of Practical Piety in John Wesley's Art of Physic." *Church History* 73, no. 4 (2004): 741–58.

Manning, Bernard Lord. *The Hymns of Wesley and Watts: Five Informal Papers*. London: Epworth Press, 1960.

Marini, Stephen. "Hymnody as History: Early Evangelical Hymns and the Recovery of American Popular Religion." *Church History* 71, no. 2 (2002): 273–307.

Marshall, Madeleine Forell, and Janet Todd. *English Congregational Hymns in the Eighteenth Century*. Lexington: University Press of Kentucky, 1982.

Maser, Frederick E. *The Story of John Wesley's Sisters, or Seven Sisters in Search of Love*. Rutland, Vermont: Academy Books, 1988.

McGonigle, Herbert Boyd. *Sufficient Saving Grace: John Wesley's Evangelical Arminianism*. Carlisle, Cumbria: Paternoster Press, 2001.

McGowen, Randall. "The Body and Punishment in Eighteenth-Century England." *The Journal of Modern History* 59, no. 4 (1987): 651–79.

McGrath, Alister E. *Christian Theology: An Introduction*. Oxford: Blackwell, 1994.

Mitchell, T. Crichton. *Charles Wesley: Man with the Dancing Heart*. Kansas City, Mo.: Beacon Hill, 1994.

Moore, Henry. *The Life of the Rev. John Wesley, A.M., Fellow of Lincoln College, Oxford: in which are included the life of his brother, the Rev. Charles Wesley, A.M., student of Christ Church, and memoirs of their family*. New York: N. Bangs and J. Emory for the Methodist Episcopal Church, 1824–25.

Morris, David B. *The Culture of Pain*. Berkeley and Los Angeles: University of California Press, 1991.

Mouw, Richard J., and Mark A. Noll, eds. *Wonderful Words of Life: Hymns in American Protestant History and Theology*. Grand Rapids, Mich.: William B. Eerdmans, 2004.

Mullan, John. *Sentiment and Sociability: The Language of Feeling in the Eighteenth Century*. Oxford: Clarendon Press, 1988.

Newport, Kenneth. "Charles Wesley's Interpretation of Some Biblical Prophecies according to a Previously Unpublished Letter Dated 25 April 1754." *Bulletin of the John Rylands University Library of Manchester* 77 (1995): 31–52.

———, ed. *The Sermons of Charles Wesley: A Critical Edition with Introduction and Notes*. Oxford: Oxford University Press, 2001.

Newport, Kenneth, and Gareth Lloyd. "George Bell and Early Methodist Enthusiasm: A New Manuscript Source from the Manchester Archives." *Bulletin of the John Rylands University Library of Manchester* 80, no. 1 (1998): 89–102.

Newport, Kenneth, and Ted A. Campbell, eds. *Charles Wesley: Life, Literature and Legacy*. Peterborough: Epworth, 2007.

Newton, John A. *Susanna Wesley and the Puritan Tradition in Methodism*. London: Epworth Press, 2002.

Noll, Mark A. *The Rise of Evangelicalism: The Age of Edwards, Whitefield and the Wesleys*. Downers Grove, Ill.: Inter-Varsity Press, 2003.

———, ed. *God and Mammon: Protestants, Money, and the Market, 1790–1860*. Oxford: Oxford University Press, 2002.

Noll, Mark A., David W. Bebbington, and George A. Rawlyk, eds. *Evangelicalism: Comparative Studies of Popular Protestantism in North America, the British Isles and Beyond, 1700–1790*. Oxford: Oxford University Press, 1994.

O'Brien, Susan. "A Transatlantic Community of Saints: The Great Awakening and the First Evangelical Network, 1735–1755." *American Historical Review* 91, no. 4 (1986): 811–32.

Olleson, Philip, ed. *The Letters of Samuel Wesley: Professional and Social Correspondence, 1797–1837*. Oxford: Oxford University Press, 2001.

Podmore, Colin. *The Moravian Church in England, 1728–1760*. Oxford: Clarendon Press, 1995.

Porter, Roy. "Pain and Suffering." Page 1575 in *Companion Encyclopedia of the History of Medicine*, edited by W. F. Bynum and Roy Porter. London: Routledge, 1993.

———. "Religion and Medicine." Pages 1449–467 in *Companion Encyclopedia of the History of Medicine*, edited by W.F. Bynum and Roy Porter. London: Routledge, 1993.

Rack, Henry D. "Evangelical Endings: Death-Beds in Evangelical Biography." *Bulletin of the John Rylands University Library of Manchester* 74, no. 1 (1992): 39–56.

———. *Reasonable Enthusiast: John Wesley and the Rise of Methodism*. Third ed. London: Epworth Press, 2002.

Rattenbury, J. Ernest. *The Eucharistic Hymns of John and Charles Wesley*. London: Epworth Press, 1948.

Reddy, William M. "Against Constructionism: The Historical Ethnography of Emotions." *Current Anthropology* 38, no. 3 (June 1997): 327–51.

Rogal, Samuel J. *John and Charles Wesley*. Boston: Twayne Publishers, 1983.

Ross, Ellen M. *The Grief of God: Images of the Suffering Jesus in Late Medieval England*. New York: Oxford University Press, 1997.

Rousseau, George Sebastian, Miranda Gill, David Haycock, and Malte Herwig, eds. *Framing and Imagining Disease in Cultural History*. Basingstoke, Hampshire: Palgrave Macmillan, 2003.

Scarry, Elaine. *The Body in Pain: The Making and Unmaking of the World*. Oxford: Oxford University Press, 1985.

Schmidt, Leigh Eric. *Hearing Things: Religion, Illusion, and the American Enlightenment*. Cambridge, Mass., and London: Harvard University Press, 2000.

Schneider, A. Gregory. *The Way of the Cross Leads Home: The Domestication of American Methodism*. Bloomington and Indianapolis: Indiana University Press, 1993.

Shields, Kenneth D. "Charles Wesley as Poet." In *Charles Wesley: Poet and Theologian*, edited by S. T. Kimbrough. Nashville: Abingdon Press, 1992.

Shoemaker, Robert B. *Gender in English Society, 1650–1850: Men and Women, Separate Spheres?* London, New York: Longman, 1989.

Shuttleton, David. "A Culture of Disfigurement: Imagining Smallpox in the Long Eighteenth Century." Pages 68–91 in *Framing and Imagining Disease in Cultural History*, edited by George Sebastian Rousseau, Miranda Gill, David Haycock, and Malte Herwig. Basingstoke, Hampshire: Palgrave Macmillan, 2003.

Smith, J. R. *The Speckled Monster: Smallpox in England, 1670–1970, With Particular Reference to Essex*. Chelmsford: Essex Records Office, 1987.

Stoddard Holmes, Martha, and Tod Chambers. "Thinking through Pain." *Literature and Medicine* 24, no. 1 (2005): 127–41.

Tarnke, Susan S. *Make a Joyful Noise unto the Lord*. Ohio: Ohio University Press, 1978.

Telford, John. *The Life of the Rev. Charles Wesley, M.A.* London: Wesleyan Methodist Book Room, 1900.

Thompson, E. P. *The Making of the English Working Class*. London: Penguin Books, 1980.

Todd, Janet. *Sensibility: An Introduction.* London, New York: Methuen, 1986.

Tyson, John R. *Charles Wesley on Sanctification: A Biographical and Theological Study*. Grand Rapids: Francis Asbury Press, 1986.

Tyson, John R. "Charles Wesley's Theology of the Cross: An Examination of the Theology and Method of Charles Wesley as Seen in His Doctrine of the Atonement." PhD diss., Drew University, 1983.

Tyson, John R. "Charles Wesley's Theology of Redemption: A Study in Structure and Method." *Wesleyan Theological Journal* 20, no. 1 (1985): 7-29.

Von Noppen, Pierre. *Transforming Words: The Early Methodist Revival from a Discourse Perspective*. Bern: Peter Lang, 1999.

Walsh, John. "John Wesley and the Community of Goods." In *Protestant Evangelicalism: Britain, Ireland, Germany and America c.1750–c.1950*, edited by Keith Robbins. Oxford: Basil Blackwell, 1990.

———. "'Methodism' and the Origins of English-Speaking Evangelicalism." Pages 19–37 in *Evangelicalism: Comparative Studies of Popular Protestantism in North America, the British Isles, and Beyond, 1700–1990*, edited by Mark A. Noll, David W. Bebbington, and George A. Rawlyk. New York, Oxford: Oxford University Press, 1994.

Ward, W. R. "The Evangelical Revival in Eighteenth-Century Britain." Pages 252–74 in *A History of Religion in Britain: Practice and Belief from the Pre-Roman Times to the Present*, edited by Sheridan Gilley and W. J. Sheils. Oxford: Blackwell, 1994.

———. *The Protestant Evangelical Awakening*. Cambridge: Cambridge University Press, 1992.

Watson, J. R., ed. *An Annotated Anthology of Hymns*. Oxford: Oxford University Press, 2002.

———. *The English Hymn: A Critical and Historical Study*. Oxford: Clarendon Press, 1997.

Whitehead, John. *The Life of the Rev. Charles Wesley: Late Student of the Christ Church, Oxford, Collected from his Private Journal*, 1793.

Wigger, John H. *Taking Heaven by Storm: Methodism and the Rise of Popular Christianity in America*. New York, Oxford: Oxford University Press, 1998.

Wise Bauer, Susan. "Stories and Syllogisms: Protestant Hymns, Narrative Theology, and Heresy." Pages 205–33 in *Wonderful Words of Life: Hymns in American Protestant History and Theology*, edited by Richard J. Mouw and Mark A. Noll. Grand Rapids, Mich.: William B. Eerdmans, 2004.

Wiseman, F. Luke. *Charles Wesley: Evangelist and Poet*. London: Epworth Press, 1932.

Woodruff, Jennifer Lynn. "John Calvin, the Wesleys and John Williamson Nevin on the Lord's Supper." *Methodist History* 41, no. 4 (2003): 159–78.

Index

About the Author

Joanna Cruickshank is a lecturer in History at Deakin University, Australia. She holds degrees in History from the Universities of Queensland and Melbourne. Her PhD dissertation, which examined the construction of suffering in the hymns of Charles Wesley, was awarded the Wesleyan Theological Society's Outstanding Dissertation Award for 2008. She has published articles and book chapters on the hymns of Charles Wesley, the autobiographical writings of early Methodist women and nineteenth-century missions in Australia.

www.ingramcontent.com/pod-product-compliance
Ingram Content Group UK Ltd.
Pitfield, Milton Keynes, MK11 3LW, UK
UKHW041102150926
475561UK00001BA/7